# Viruses and Human Cancer

*Edited by*

## *J.R. Arrand*[a] *and D.R. Harper*[b]

[a]Paterson Institute for Cancer Research, Christie Hospital,
Manchester M20 4BX, UK

*and*

[b]Department of Virology, St Bartholomew's and the Royal London School of
Medicine and Dentistry, London EC1A 7BE, UK

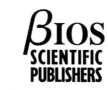

*β*IOS
SCIENTIFIC
PUBLISHERS

Oxford • Washington DC

© BIOS Scientific Publishers Limited, 1998

Copyright held by BIOS Scientific Publishers Ltd. for all chapters except that on page 39.

First published 1998

A CIP catalogue record for this book is available from the British Library.

ISBN 1-8727-844-9

BIOS Scientific Publishers Ltd
9 Newtec Place, Magdalen Road, Oxford OX4 1RE, UK
Tel. +44 (0)1865 726286. Fax +44 (0)1865 246823
World Wide Web home page: http://www.bios.co.uk

DISTRIBUTORS

*Australia and New Zealand*
   Blackwell Science Asia
   54 University Street
   Carlton, South Victoria 3053

*India*
   Viva Books Private Limited
   4325/3 Ansari Road, Daryaganj
   New Delhi 110002

*Singapore and South East Asia*
   APAC Publishers Services
   Block 12 Lorong Bakar Batu #05-09
   Kolam Ayer Industrial Estate
   Singapore 348745

*USA and Canada*
   BIOS Scientific Publishers
   PO Box 605, Herndon
   VA 20172-0605

Production Editor: Andrea Bosher.
Typeset by Banbury Graphics Ltd, Banbury, UK.
Printed by Biddles Ltd, Guildford, UK.

# Contents

# Abbreviations

| | |
|---|---|
| Ad | adenovirus |
| AFP | alpha-fetoprotein |
| AIDS-KS | AIDS-related Kaposi's sarcoma |
| ALL | acute lymphoblastic leukaemia |
| ATLL | adult T-cell leukaemia/lymphoma |
| ATLV | adult T-cell leukaemia virus |
| BL | Burkitt's lymphoma |
| BLV | bovine leukaemia virus |
| BPV | bovine papillomavirus |
| CAT | chloramphenicol acetyl transferase |
| ccc | covalently closed circular (genome) |
| CCT | cytoplasmic carboxyl terminus |
| cdk | cyclin-dependent kinase |
| CHO | Chinese hamster ovary (cell line) |
| $CID_{50}$ | chimpanzee infectious dose$_{50}$ |
| CIN | cervical intraepithelial neoplasia/dysplasia |
| CIS | carcinoma *in situ* |
| CMV | cytomegalovirus |
| CR1,CR2 | conserved region 1,2 |
| CRE | cyclic AMP-responsive element |
| CRPV | cottontail rabbit papillomavirus |
| CTL | cytotoxic T lymphocyte |
| E6-AP | E6-associated protein |
| EA | Epstein–Barr virus early antigen |
| EBNA | Epstein–Barr virus nuclear antigen |
| EBV | Epstein–Barr virus |
| EGF | epidermal growth factor |
| EIAV | equine infectious anaemia virus |
| EV | epidermodysplasia verruciformis |
| GPCR | G-protein-coupled receptor |
| GST | glutathione-S-transferase |
| HAM | HTLV-1-associated myelopathy |
| HBcAg | hepatitis B virus core antigen |
| HBeAg | hepatitis B virus soluble/secretory protein |
| HBIG | hepatitis B immune globulin |
| HBsAg | hepatitis B virus surface antigen |
| HBV | hepatitis B virus |
| HCC | hepatocellular carcinoma |

| | |
|---|---|
| HCL | hairy cell leukaemia |
| HCV | hepatitis C virus |
| HD | Hodgkin's disease |
| HFV | human foamy virus |
| HHV-8 | human herpesvirus 8 |
| HLA | human leucocyte antigen |
| HPV | human papillomavirus |
| HSV | herpes simplex virus |
| HTLV | human T-cell leukaemia virus/ T-lymphotropic virus |
| IFN | interferon |
| IL | interleukin |
| IL-2R | interleukin-2 receptor |
| IM | infectious mononucleosis |
| IVDU | intravenous drug user |
| KS | Kaposi's sarcoma |
| KSHV | Kaposi's sarcoma-associated virus |
| LCL | lymphoblastoid cell line |
| LCR | long control region |
| LMP | Epstein–Barr virus latent membrane protein |
| LP | leader protein |
| LT | large T antigen |
| LTR | long terminal repeat |
| MA | Epstein–Barr virus membrane antigen |
| MDV | Marek's disease virus |
| MHC | major histocompatibility complex |
| MIP | macrophage inflammatory protein |
| MLV | murine leukaemia virus |
| MMTV | mouse mammary tumour virus |
| NDV | Newcastle disease virus |
| NK | natural killer |
| NPC | nasopharyngeal carcinoma |
| OHL | oral hairy leukoplakia |
| ORF | open reading frame |
| PBMC | peripheral blood mononuclear cell |
| PCNA | proliferating cell nuclear antigen |
| PCR | polymerase chain reaction |
| PDGF | platelet-derived growth factor |
| pRB | retinoblastoma susceptibility gene product |
| RB | retinoblastoma |
| *RB-1* | retinoblastoma gene |
| RBP-Jκ | human Jκ recombination signal sequence binding protein |
| RS | Reed-Sternberg |
| RSV | Rous sarcoma virus |
| RT | reverse transcriptase |
| SCID | severe combined immune deficiency |

| STLV | simian T-cell lymphotropic virus |
| SV40 | simian virus 40 |
| TBP | TATA-binding protein |
| TCR | T-cell receptor |
| TNFR | tumour necrosis factor receptor |
| TPA | 12-O-tetradacanoylphorbol-13-acetate |
| TRAF | tumour necrosis factor receptor associated factor |
| TSP | Tropical spastic paraparesis |
| u.v. | ultraviolet |
| VCA | Epstein–Barr virus capsid antigen |
| VDEPT | virus-directed enzyme/prodrug therapy |
| vIL10 | Epstein–Barr virus IL-10 (interleukin) homologue |
| vIL-6 | viral interleukin-6 |
| VLP | virus-like particle |
| VZV | varicella-zoster virus |
| WHV | woodchuck hepatitis virus |
| XLP | X-linked lymphoproliferative syndrome |
| XP | xeroderma pigmentosum |

# Contributors

**Arrand, J.R.,** *Paterson Institute for Cancer Research, Christie Hospital NHS Trust, Manchester, M20 4BX, UK*

**Harper, D.R.,** *Department of Virology, St. Bartholomew's and the Royal London School of Medicine and Dentistry, London, EC1A 7BE, UK*

**Harrison, T.J.,** *University Department of Medicine, Royal Free Hospital School of Medicine, London, NW3 2PF, UK*

**McClure, M.,** *Department of Genito-Urinary Medicine and Communicable Diseases, Imperial College School of Medicine at St. Mary's, London W2 1PG, UK*

**Phillips, A.C.,** *ABL Basic Research Program, NCI-FCRDC Building 560, Room 22–96, West 7th Street, Frederick, MD 21702, USA*

**Smith, N.A.,** *Institute of Cancer Research, Chester Beatty Laboratories, London SW3 6JB, UK*

**Talbot, S.J.,** *Institute of Cancer Research, Chester Beatty Laboratories, London SW3 6JB, UK*

**Taylor, G.P.,** *Department of Genito-Urinary Medicine and Communicable Diseases, Imperial College School of Medicine at St. Mary's, London W2 1PG, UK*

**Vousden, K.H.,** *ABL Basic Research Program, NCI-FCRDC Building 560, Room 22–96, West 7th Street, Frederick, MD 21702, USA*

**Weiss, R.A.,** *Institute of Cancer Research, Chester Beatty Laboratories, London SW3 6JB, UK*

**Whitby, D.,** *Institute of Cancer Research, Chester Beatty Laboratories, London SW3 6JB, UK*

# Preface

"Because experimental and epidemiologic data imply a causative role for viruses, particularly in cervical and liver cancer, viruses must be thought of as the second most important risk factor for cancer development in humans, exceeded only by tobacco consumption" [1].

Although it has been long considered likely that viruses have a role in human tumorigenesis it is only relatively recently that sufficient evidence has been amassed to enable zur Hausen's statement to be made with authority. It is now clear that five virus types are involved in the causation of human cancer: papillomaviruses, retroviruses, herpesviruses, hepadnaviruses and flaviviruses. Each of these is considered in depth in the chapters which follow.

Tumour virology has a long history and, using model systems, has been the source of much of our fundamental knowledge of oncogenesis and basic cellular mechanisms (e.g. oncogenes were discovered in avian retroviruses, mRNA splicing was first described in human adenoviruses). Some of this rich history is revisited in the first chapter.

Enthusiasm for tumour virology remains high and the search for new agents continues. A recent detailed epidemiological study failed to provide evidence for hitherto unknown oncogenic viruses [2] but this disappointment was tempered by the exciting discovery, using a new molecular technique, of a new herpesvirus implicated in the genesis of Kaposi's sarcoma [3]. Tumour virology is still an exciting area: e.g. molecular mechanisms of virus-induced cellular transformation are being unravelled, EBV is implicated in an increasing variety of neoplasms, vaccine strategies to prevent virus-induced cancer are showing success and novel therapeutic strategies are being developed.

There is still much to be understood. It is hoped that this little book will whet the appetites of a new generation of tumour virologists.

J.R. Arrand
D.R. Harper

## References

1. **Zur Hausen, H.** (1991) *Science* **254:** 1167–1173.
2. **Memon, A. and Doll, R.** (1994) *Int. J. Cancer* **58:** 366-368.
3. **Chang, Y., Cesarman, E., Pessin, M.S., Lee, F., Culpepper, J., Knowles, D.M. and Moore, P.S.** (1994) *Science* **266:** 1865–1869.

Chapter 1

# Introducing viruses and cancer

## Robin A. Weiss

## 1.1 Importance

Oncogenic viruses are important for two main reasons. First, approximately 15% of human cancer incidence can be attributed to virus infection. A major proportion of these infections may one day be prevented by immunization (see Chapter 7), significantly lowering the worldwide cancer burden. Second, the experimental study of tumour viruses in animals and humans has illuminated cancer more generally. For example, oncogenes and tumour suppressor genes were first identified through studies of tumour viruses.

## 1.2 Flashback on viral carcinogenesis

The first human tumour virus, Epstein–Barr virus (EBV) was discovered in 1964 in Burkitt's lymphoma cells by Epstein, Achong and Barr. Later, EBV was also detected in a form of undifferentiated nasopharyngeal carcinoma (see Chapter 4). Infectious hepatitis was suspected of being linked to liver cancer since the 1940s, but until hepatitis B virus (HBV) was discovered and viral markers became available, the virus could not be firmly linked with the cancer (see Chapter 2). In fact, it was Beaseley's epidemiological, prospective study of men with HBV infection in Taiwan that confirmed the association. Today, the link between another hepatitis virus (HCV) and liver cancer remains solely epidemiological, though the evidence is gaining strength.

In 1980, Gallo discovered human T-cell leukaemia virus (HTLV-I) and it soon became linked with adult T-cell leukaemia in Japan by Miyoshi and Hinuma and in the West Indies by Catovsky (see Chapter 6). Human papillomavirus (HPV) strains 16 and 18 were discovered only in 1983 by zur Hausen and colleagues through techniques of molecular hybridization in cancer of the uterine cervix (see Chapter 3) although as early as the 19th century

*Viruses and Human Cancer*, edited by J.R. Arrand and D.R. Harper
© 1998 BIOS Scientific Publishers Ltd, Oxford

1

cervical cancer was postulated to be sexually transmissible. Kaposi's sarcoma (KS) was thought to have an infectious aetiology for many decades, yet the apparent culprit – human herpes virus 8 (HHV-8) – only came to light 3 years ago (see Chapter 5).

Viruses and cancer, however, have a longer history in animal studies. Leukaemia in chickens was experimentally transmitted by "an agent that passed through a filter" by Danish researchers in 1908 and soon afterwards Peyton Rous, in New York, showed the same for chicken sarcoma. The medical research community was not receptive to the notion of transmissible cancer, and eventually Rous became disillusioned. Happily, he lived to be awarded the Nobel Prize in 1966, 55 years after his great discovery. Two further Nobel Awards in Medicine came through studies of Rous sarcoma virus (RSV): to Howard Temin and David Baltimore in 1975 for their 1970 discovery of reverse transcriptase, and to Harold Varmus and Michael Bishop in 1989 for showing in 1976 that the *src* oncogene of RSV-transformed cells was derived from a cellular gene.

Laboratory mice, too, have played an important role in our understanding of viral cancers. In 1936 Bittner showed that predisposition to breast cancer in C3H mice was passed through the milk to their offspring. By foster-nursing C3H baby mice on low incidence C67Black mothers, he broke the chain of transmission, and by fostering C57Blacks on C3H mothers they became susceptible to breast cancer. The 'milk factor' was later shown to be the mouse mammary tumour virus (MMTV), a retrovirus. The development of the cancer is hormone-dependent, and the virus itself is stimulated by glucocorticoid and oestrogenic steroids. After infant mice take the virus up through the gut, MMTV infects B lymphocytes. It stimulates their proliferation by encoding a protein that acts as a superantigen. Only after puberty and during pregnancy does the virus colonize mammary epithelial cells. In one strain of mouse, GR, Multbock found that breast cancer predisposition is inherited genetically as a Mendelian dominant trait. But this too turned out to be a strain of MMTV, in this case passed as an integrated DNA provirus in the chromosomes of the germ line. This proved to be an early example of what are now called endogenous retroviruses.

As with breast cancer, murine lymphoma depends on retroviruses and host genes. In the 1930s Jacob Furth began inbreeding mice selecting for a 'high leukaemia strain'. These AKR mice develop thymic T-cell lymphomas at a relatively early age. In 1951 Ludwig Gross found that the tumour cells release a virus that transmits the propensity for lymphoma to C3H mice. We now know that this is one of the murine leukaemia viruses (MLV), belonging to the retrovirus family. MLV strains have been studied extensively in experimental oncogenesis; they also form the basis of retroviral vectors for gene therapy (see Section 7.7).

Gross' early studies were confusing because some mice developed multiple types of carcinoma as well as lymphoma. Eventually he discovered that he was transmitting a mixture of viruses. MLV, which has a lipid envelope, was sensitive to inactivation by lipid solvents such as ether; the virus causing carcinomas was ether resistant and it was isolated independently in 1958 by Stewart and Eddy and was named polyoma virus. This was one of the first small DNA tumour viruses to be studied, although Richard Shope had studied skin cancer induced by papillomaviruses in rabbits in the 1930s.

In 1960, a cytopathic virus was observed by Maurice Hilleman in monkey kidney cultures used for the propagation of polio virus for the Salk (killed) and Sabin (live–attenuated) vaccines. Monolayer culture and cell trypsinization were still relatively novel techniques, yet it was immediately apparent that this 'vacuolating' virus called SV40 (simian virus 40) was present in polio vaccine preparations. Between 1955 and 1963 some 200 million people may have been exposed to SV40-contaminated vaccines. Recently, claims have been made that certain human tumours, such as mesothelioma and paediatric central nervous system tumours (ependemona, choroid plexus tumour) contain SV40 sequences as detected by the polymerase chain reaction. At the time of writing, these findings remain controversial, because SV40 DNA sequences are often present in laboratory reagents such as plasmids which might yield false-positive results. Nevertheless, Hilleman's original investigations had shown that SV40 was highly oncogenic in hamsters and other rodents, often inducing the same types of tumour which investigators now think it is present in humans. The SV40-positive human brain tumours, however, come from children born long after polio vaccines were cleaned up, so if the results are confirmed, it implies that SV40 is transmitted between humans.

The discovery of polyoma virus and SV40 opened up the field of DNA tumour viruses. These viruses have small genomes with only one to three proteins (the T or tumour antigens) expressed in non-productive, neoplastically transformed rodent cells. The human viruses, BK and JC (named after the initials of the patients from whom they were originally isolated) are related to SV40. They are also oncogenic in hamsters but not, apparently, in humans. The ability of polyoma virus, SV40 and Rous sarcoma virus to transform fibroblasts in culture greatly hastened the study of viral transforming genes. Renato Dulbecco was awarded the Nobel Prize in 1975 (alongside Temin and Baltimore) for pioneering the field of *in vitro* neoplastic transformation by oncogenic viruses. Later, in 1979, cellular p53 protein was discovered through its co-precipitation with SV40 large T antigen by Linzer and Levine in the USA and by Lane and Crawford in the UK. These days, where yeast two-hybrid systems are routine in research laboratories, protein–protein interactions seem commonplace, but less than 20 years ago the idea that a viral protein could become specifically coupled with a cellular protein and thereby altered cellular function was quite novel.

Just as bacteriophages opened up molecular biology and genetics in the 1950s the study of animal viruses, especially oncogenic viruses, has led to fundamental insights into the molecular biology of eukaryotic cells. For example, it was through the study of the transforming genes of SV40 and adenovirus that Philip Sharp observed that mRNA mapped to two non-contiguous parts of the viral genome. This was the first discovery of RNA splicing and it led to another Nobel prize.

Domestic animals have also revealed oncogenic viruses at work. Pox viruses in rabbits were shown to cause skin tumours by Shope in 1933. Most pox viruses are not oncogenic although the pox virus that causes human molluscum contagiosum does induce a benign proliferative disease. Pox viruses contain several genes homologous to cellular genes some of which are mitogenic. A retrovirus similar to MLV causing leukaemia in cats was discovered in 1964 and cattle harbour a retrovirus more closely related to HTLV-I. This became widely endemic, spreading via the veterinarians needle, when cattle were immunized against other microbes, reminiscent of the iatrogenic (doctor-caused) spread of human immunodeficiency virus (HIV) two decades later through contaminated blood and blood products. Cattle also have papillomaviruses, which have proved useful both in studying cell transformation and as viral vectors. In addition to retroviruses causing leukaemia, chickens suffer from a transmissible lymphoma called Marek's disease that frequently invades nerves. Marek's disease virus (MDV) is a herpesvirus discovered in 1967. Together with EBV, MDV provided a model for studying lymphomagenic herpesviruses more generally. New world monkeys also have lymphomagenic herpesviruses, and several species of fish are infected with lymphomagenic retroviruses. Thus, many kinds of vertebrate, from fish to man, play host to oncogenic viruses.

## 1.3 Human tumour virus epidemiology

Human cancer is not commonly thought to be 'catching'. Indeed, even with those cancers that have a viral aetiology, it is unusual to view cancer as contagious. This is because cancer is an infrequent consequence of infection by the causative virus and often occurs years after the initial infection has taken place. Thus, the virus may be generally present in the human population, for example EBV, or may be prevalent in a significant proportion of healthy people in endemic areas, for example HTLV–I and KS–associated herpes virus (KSHV/HHV-8).

*Table 1.1* lists the known human viruses with oncogenic potential. Among them are some human viruses that are highly oncogenic in experimental animals and yet are not linked epidemiologically with human cancer at all. Some adenoviruses fall into this category as do the human polyoma viruses, BK and JC. It may, in some circumstances, be as relevant to investigate why these viruses do not cause human cancer as to explain why others do. Does the immune system stop them exerting an oncogenic effect or is their replication and gene expression different in their natural and experimental hosts? Similar examples exist among animals. For example, herpesvirus saimiri is closely related to HHV-8, and is also related to EBV. It appears to be harmless in its natural host, the squirrel monkey, but it is highly oncogenic in other new world primates such as the owl monkey. However, it is not known whether it might

**Table 1.1.** Human viruses with oncogenic potential

| | Virus | Human tumours | Non-malignant disease | Experimental tumours in animals |
|---|---|---|---|---|
| *Papovaviridae* | Human papillomavirus | Cervical cancer Skin cancer | Warts | |
| | BK | None | Not known | Multiple tumours in rodents |
| | JC | None | Progressive multifocal leukoencephalopathy | Multiple tumours in rodents |
| *Adenoviridae* | Adenovirus | None | Gut and respiratory infections | Sarcomas, carcinomas in rodents |
| *Herpesviridae* | Epstein–Barr virus | Nasopharyngeal carcinoma Burkitt's lymphoma Immunoblastic lymphoma Hodgkin's lymphoma | Infectious mononucleosis | Lymphoma in monkeys |
| | Human herpesvirus 8 | Kaposi's sarcoma Primary effusion lymphoma | Multicentric Castleman's disease | Not known |
| *Retroviridae* | HTLV-1[a] | Adult T-cell leukaemia | Tropical spastic paraparesis | ATL[c] in rabbits |
| | HIV[b] (indirect) | B-cell lymphoma Kaposi's sarcoma | AIDS[d] | |
| *Hepadnaviridae* | Hepatitis B virus | Liver cancer | Hepatitis Cirrhosis | Not known |
| *Flaviviridae* | Hepatitis C virus (indirect) | Liver cancer | Hepatitis Cirrhosis | Not known |

[a] Human T-cell leukaemia virus.
[b] Human immune deficiency virus.
[c] Adult T-cell leukaemia.
[d] Acquired immune deficiency syndrome.

occasionally be oncogenic in its natural host, as EBV is in humans, because only small numbers of squirrel monkeys have been studied.

One reason why cancer is a rare consequence of infection by oncogenic viruses may be that the viruses are insufficient in themselves to cause full malignancy. Epidemiologists have estimated from the age incidences of non-viral cancers that four to six causal, independent events are required to induce human malignancy. Studies of the molecular genetics of human cancer suggest that these events are mainly mutations. The likelihood of clocking up so many oncogenic mutations in a single clonal cell lineage is small and hence cancer is rare on a cellular basis. Moreover, deleterious mutations of tumour suppressor genes tend to be recessive. As each adult human has approximately $10^{14}$ cells at any time and in some tissues there is rapid renewal of cells from stem cells, cancer has an increasing chance of developing with age. A familial predisposition to cancer usually means that just one of the genetic changes is inherited from one of the parents, such as RB in familial retinoblastoma and p53 in Li–Fraumeni syndrome. Infection by a tumour virus represents the equivalent of just one or two of the steps that would occur by mutation, although the virus will be present in perhaps millions of cells and therefore should increase the probability of cancer development considerably. However, as discussed later, cell mediated immunity against virus-infected cells will decrease their probability of emerging as fully cancerous cells.

Given the multistep nature of carcinogenesis, the virus may be a necessary step but alone might not cause the cancer. Several examples of the multistage process of viral carcinogenesis can be cited.

***Burkitt's lymphoma (BL).*** (See Section 4.8.3) This is a rare B-cell lymphoma that occurs sporadically in adults across the world. However, it also occurs at much higher frequency in young children in areas of holoendemic infection by falciparum malaria. In almost every case of endemic children's BL, EBV is present in the lymphoma cells; but EBV is rarely present in adult BL. What is common to both children's and adult BL is a t8;14 chromosome translocation that brings the c-*myc* cellular oncogene on chromosome 8 under the control of the immunoglobulin heavy chain gene promoter (in about 20% of BL the c-*myc* gene is translocated to loci on chromosomes 2 or 22 adjacent to the genes for the kappa and lambda immunoglobulin light chains). So what actually causes BL? The *myc* translocation is a paramount feature and occurs independently of EBV infection, probably at a later stage of oncogenesis. We know that EBV can lead infected B cells to proliferate indefinitely in culture, a process known as immortalization. But as more than 80% of the human population becomes infected by EBV in infancy why is BL restricted to children repeatedly infected by malaria? It used to be thought that malaria caused immunodeficiency. In fact the immune dysregulation most likely to be directly associated with the development of BL is enhanced proliferation of B cells. This may allow EBV to expand its targets for infection and to extend its immortalizing effect.

***Primary liver cancer.*** (See Chapter 2). Although primary hepatocellular carcinoma is rare in the west, it is common in Africa and Asia. Both HBV and HCV are independently associated with liver cancer. While the relative risk of developing liver cancer upon chronic infection with HBV is only about four-fold, in many HBV endemic areas the actual risk of liver cancer is about 80-fold greater than in western populations. The reason for this large discrepancy is likely to be the interaction with another liver carcinogen, aflatoxin. Aflatoxins are products of certain moulds that grow on foodstuffs such as ground nuts and cereals stored in hot, humid climates. Aflatoxin acts as a strong liver carcinogen when fed to rats. As with HBV, humans who regularly eat aflatoxin-contaminated food appear to have approximately a four-fold increased incidence of liver cancer. But HBV-infected people who are also exposed to aflatoxin may exhibit the higher, 80-fold risk, for example in parts of West Africa and in Mozambique. Thus, the viral and the dietary carcinogens appear to act synergistically, one exacerbating the effect of the other. How this might occur will be discussed under general mechanisms of carcinogenesis.

*Skin cancer in epidermodysplasia verruciformis (EV).* (See also Section 3.2). EV is an extremely rare single gene recessive disorder that gives rise to multiple warts (papillomas) all over the body. Where the skin of EV patients is exposed to sunlight, malignant squamous carcinoma often develops in addition to benign warts. The ultraviolet (uv) radiation in sunlight acts as a carcinogen to which EV sufferers are particularly sensitive, as in patients with inherited xeroderma pigmentosum (xp). Where EV differs from XP is that certain human papillomaviruses (HPV-5, -8 and related genomes) are found in EV tumours. The recessive heritable defect predisposes the HPV to form warts which, when exposed to uv light, often convert to malignancy.

Thus, the two environmental carcinogens, HPV and uv radiation act together to cause the malignancy, but this risk is enormously higher in EV patients than in normal individuals. In fact until recently, HPV-5 and HPV-8 had not been detected in people without EV. Because the chance of HPV transmitting from one EV patient to another is minuscule, it seemed likely that there must be intermediate human hosts. These have now come to light, partly due to the sensitivity of the polymerase chain reaction (PCR) detection system, but mainly in immunosuppressed subjects. Recipients of organ transplants, who are immunosuppressed as part of their treatment, have an increased risk of squamous skin cancers, and these tumours carry HPV-5 or it relatives. Patients with acquired immune deficiency syndrome (AIDS) also sometimes present with HPV-5-containing warts, although invasive skin cancer is less common in this form of immune suppression than in transplant recipients.

## 1.4 Immune surveillance and viral carcinogenesis

In 1909 Paul Ehrlich suggested that but for the immune system, cancer would occur much more commonly. He proposed that the increase in cancer among the elderly was a consequence of impaired immune responses, especially what we today call cell-mediated immunity. The immune surveillance theory of cancer was further developed by McFarlane Burnett and Lewis Thomas in the 1950s. It remains popular today, particularly among proponents of alternative and complementary medicine.

Despite the acceptance of immune surveillance against cancer, there is little evidence to support it, except for viral cancers. The evidence against general immune surveillance keeping cancer at bay comes from an examination of cancer incidence in immunodeficient conditions. Mice that are immuno-suppressed or are bred to be immune deficient [e.g. nude mice and those with severe combined immune deficiency (SCID)] are more susceptible to certain kinds of cancer, but not to all cancers generally. The increase in cancer is associated mainly with infection by retroviruses or by other oncogenic viruses, for example polyoma virus. Two recent human conditions of T-cell immune deficiency have also yielded valuable insight to the immune surveillance theory of cancer. They are iatrogenically immunosuppressed recipients of allo-geneic organs and tissues, and patients with AIDS. These subjects also demonstrate that while there is a high relative risk for some viral cancers, the common cancers of the bowel, breast, squamous carcinoma of the lung, etc. are not markedly increased.

The most common cancers of immunodeficient patients are B-cell lymphoma (mainly associated with EBV; see Section 4.8.4) and KS (associated with HHV-8; see Chapter 5). In addition there is a more modest relative risk of cervical carcinoma, and of anal carcinoma in homosexuals (HPV-16, -18-type viruses). There is also some evidence of an increase in skin cancer caused by HPV, lung cancer and germ cell cancer of the testes and the epidemiological evidence suggests that it might be worthwhile to seek to associate viruses with these cancers. Certainly the enormous increase in KS in homosexual men with AIDS gave renewed impetus to identify the virus associated with this disease.

Why should only viral cancers be at higher risk in immunodeficient humans or mice? Probably the answer is that in the majority of these tumours, viral antigens persist and are recognized as foreign, whereas no foreign anti-gens are present in cancers arising by non-infectious processes. Immunity is best understood for EBV infection (see Section 4.6). Undoubtedly, cell-mediated immunity, especially cytotoxic T lymphocytes (CTL), controls the number of EBV-infected B cells. Removal or diminution of this immune constraint can act to increase EBV-related cancers in two possible ways: by eliminating incipient cancer cells; and by reducing the overall viral load so that fewer B cells become infected by EBV at any one time. CTL responses to viral antigens expressed in latent infection, such as latent membrane protein, will control the growth of transformed cells; CTL responses to lytic antigens will kill cells that have switched into virus production before much virus is released.

It is interesting to note that the type of B-cell tumours most commonly found in immune deficiency are large, immunoblastic cell lymphomas (see Section 4.8.4), Burkitt's lymphoma cells being less frequent. Immunoblastic lymphoma resembles the non-malignant proliferative disease, infectious mononucleosis (Section 4.8.1), associated with adult or teenage primary EBV infection, except that it is not self-limiting. Duncan's syndrome (Section 4.8.6), a disease of infants who inherit a specific deficiency in mounting an immune response to EBV, also develop similar tumours. These lymphomas may initially be polyclonal in origin, as judged by the analysis of immunoglobulin gene rearrangements, but often a monoclonal neoplasm emerges.

## 1.5 General mechanisms of viral carcinogenesis

The way in which oncogenic viruses induce tumours may be viewed as two major mechanisms: direct oncogenesis means that the virus infects a progenitor of the clonal tumour cell population, and usually persists in the tumour cells; and indirect oncogenesis could occur when the virus does not necessarily infect the tumour progenitor cell, but may exert an indirect effect on cell and tissue turnover or on the immune system, which predisposes towards tumour development.

Most tumour virus research has been devoted to directly oncogenic viruses. Before turning to the molecular mechanisms by which these viruses transform cells into a neoplastic state, it is worth considering indirect viral carcinogenesis a little further.

For viruses that have an indirect effect in promoting carcinogenesis, it is difficult to obtain definitive evidence of causality. Indeed, it is difficult enough to satisfy Koch's postulates (*Table 1.2*) even with directly oncogenic viruses, considering the long 'incubation' period between initial exposure to the virus and tumour development, that tumours are not the inevitable outcome of infection, and that other factors or causes also contribute to multistep carcinogenesis. With indirect effects, the main evidence remains epidemiological, that is that there is a significantly increased risk of the cancer associated with infection by the virus. When the virus is ubiquitous, like EBV or adenoviruses, establishing an association between virus and cancer becomes unfeasible if the virus is not present in the cancer cell.

One example of indirect viral carcinogenesis, as already discussed, is of viruses that cause immune deficiency. The increased risk of KS and of B-cell lymphoma in AIDS reflects the similar increase in these tumours in patients immunosuppressed by non-viral means. Thus we may argue that HIV causes immune deficiency and that deficiency underlies the development of these cancers. HIV, then, is an indirect cause, and HHV-8 and EBV are the direct causes, respectively, of KS and B-cell lymphoma.

In multifactorial carcinogenesis, however, causes do not always fit so precisely as those just outlined. For example, whereas > 90% of B-cell lymphomas in immunosuppressed transplant patients are EBV-positive, EBV accounts for only 50% of AIDS lymphomas; we do not know whether the remaining 50% contain an unknown tumour virus, or whether the B-cell

**Table 1.2.** Koch's Postulates. In the late 1800s, the celebrated German microbiologist Robert Koch (1843–1910) formulated a set of criteria which should be fulfilled in order to associate a micro-organism as being the causative agent of a particular disease.

1. The micro-organism must be regularly found in the lesions of the disease.
2. It can be isolated in pure culture on artificial media.
3. Inoculation of this culture must produce a similar disease in experimental animals.
4. The micro-organism must be recoverable from the lesions in these animals.

hyperplasia that is a feature of HIV infection may allow expansion of B-cell clones that accumulate chromosome translocations without the need for a directly transforming virus.

For KS, a contributing effect of the *tat* gene product of HIV has been postulated. The Tat protein can be secreted from HIV-infected cells and may exert an angiogenic, proliferative effect in concert with basic fibroblast growth factor on endothelial cells, the progenitor cells of KS. There is some evidence in West Africa for a greater incidence of KS in HHV-8-positive patients who have AIDS caused by HIV-1 rather than by HIV-2. Perhaps a difference in the Tat protein of the two HIV types could account for the difference in KS incidence, though that remains entirely speculative.

Another example of possible indirect carcinogenesis concerns primary liver cancer and HCV infection (see Section 2.7.3). HCV is the only RNA virus that is associated with cancer (other than the *Retroviridae* which make DNA in the infected cells). HCV genomes are not routinely found in the cancer cells of infected liver specimens. HCV does, however, cause liver cell death and cirrhosis, calling on renewal from and proliferation of liver stem cells. If these cells are concurrently exposed to mutagens like aflatoxin as discussed earlier, then it is reasonable to interpret the 'carcinogenic' effect of HCV to result from stimulating proliferation of progenitor cells not necessarily infected by the virus. In this model the virus is analogous to the promoter effect of chemicals such as phorbol esters on cells initiated by mutagenic carcinogens.

HBV is assumed to be directly oncogenic, because the virus is found frequently in the cancer cells of primary hepatocellular carcinoma, sometimes integrated into the chromosomal DNA. However, if HCV can promote liver cancer indirectly, it is likely that HBV could have the same effect through liver cell destruction, cirrhosis and progenitor cell renewal (see Section 2.7.4). However, some other causes of cirrhosis, for example inherited Wilson's disease, are not associated with liver cancer, although alcohol-induced liver damage does present a cancer risk.

Finally, there are some malignancies in which an infectious component of their aetiology has been postulated, but in which no oncogenic virus has yet been discovered. The most important example of these is acute lymphoblastic leukaemia (ALL) in children. Although paediatric ALL is rare, it sometimes occurs in clusters. At first it was thought that these groups of cases might be linked with sources of ionizing radiation, but it now appears that there is a stronger association with population mixing, when newcomers to rural areas mix with longer established, indigenous populations. Exposure to viruses (or other infections), or perhaps delays in exposure within such isolated communities to infectious agents which are more common in areas of high population density, might account for such clusters of ALL. If this hypothesis is correct, it may be related to a specific virus, or it might be the result of immune responses to a number of different infectious agents not usually related to leukaemia. More research needs to be done to see if the model holds up and if so, whether it can be pinned down to a specific pathogen.

## 1.6 Molecular mechanisms of viral carcinogenesis

Much knowledge has accrued over the past two decades on the molecular biology of cell transformation by oncogenic viruses. Each virus differs and is discussed in the chapters devoted to those viruses. Here, it is worth commenting on the commonality of effector pathways and on how viral oncogenesis has illuminated cancer research more generally.

Cancer cells are genetically altered, and that may include the insertion of viral genes. Firstly, oncogenes may be ectopically expressed, that is, switched on; secondly, tumour suppressor genes may be inappropriately switched off; thirdly, signals that would normally switch cells into programmed cell death, apoptosis, may be diverted so that damaged cells survive to become malignant. Directly oncogenic viruses infect the precursor cells destined to become malignant, and by and large, the viral genome (or a part of it) persists in those cells. The viral genome or its gene products, viral proteins, can affect oncogenes, tumour suppressor genes and apoptotic pathways. Although viral oncogenesis is a by-product of viral replication, and a very rare one in proportion to the total number of cells infected, it can be of advantage to the virus to stimulate proliferation of its host cell, or to delay apoptosis. This is true even for viruses that are lytic late in the replication cycle. Killed cells cannot become cancer cells, of course, which is one reason why apoptosis is such a good fail-safe mechanism in normal physiology and development. However, lytic viruses with defective replication cycles can induce malignant transformation through the proliferative stimuli of their early gene products.

An example of common effector pathways is that of the small oncogenic DNA viruses. Adenovirus, polyoma virus and papillomavirus strains establish infection best in proliferating cells, even though in the case of papillomaviruses, late stages of replication only occur in post-mitotic, terminally differentiated cells. Each of these three types of virus has the capacity to inactivate the same cellular tumour suppressor proteins, namely retinoblastoma (RB) and p53 (*Table 1.3*). Viral proteins bind to p53, for example, and sequester it so that it cannot function as a check point for initiation of DNA replication or to trigger apoptosis. The viral protein–p53 complex may simply inactivate p53 function, or lead to its rapid degradation, but the final effect is the same. Similar mechanisms operate for RB.

**Table 1.3.** Tumour suppressor proteins inactivated by tumour viruses

| Host protein | Viral protein | Virus |
|---|---|---|
| RB | E1A | Adenovirus |
| | Large T | SV40, BK |
| | E7 | HPV-16, HPV-18 |
| p53 | E1B | Adenovirus |
| | Large T | SV40, BK |
| | E6 | HPV-16, HPV-18 |

With retroviruses, other mechanisms of oncogenesis operate (*Figure 1.1*). The most notorious is that they can acquire cellular oncogenes as part of their own genome. In 1911, when Peyton Rous demonstrated induction of sarcomas in chickens, we can surmise with hindsight that he actually selected an avian leukosis virus which had transduced a cellular oncogene, *src*. In fact, oncogene-bearing retroviruses are found only rarely in naturally occurring retroviral tumours, and such transducing viruses are usually defective, having swapped part of their replicative genome for the oncogene. The great majority of retroviral tumours are induced as a consequence of the integration of the DNA provirus next to a cellular proto-oncogene in the host genome. The proviral long terminal repeat (LTR) contains strong promoter and enhancer sequences and can thus switch on the cellular oncogene to cause unscheduled cell cycling. This mechanism is directly analogous to chromosome transloca-tions activating cellular oncogenes; the strong promoter of an immunoglobu-lin gene activating c-*myc* in BL is equivalent to the LTR of avian leukosis virus activating c-*myc* by insertion just upstream to it in B-cell precursors in the bursa of Fabricius.

The HTLV-I (see Chapter 6) and its relative, bovine leukosis virus, have a different mechanism of oncogenesis (*Figure 1.1*). These viruses have addi-tional genes to *gag, pol* and *env* which are universal to all retroviruses. The *tax* gene encodes a protein that transactivates transcription of viral RNA from the LTR. In other words it acts as a positive feedback signal in that a low expres-sion of Tax protein stimulates further viral gene expression. Tax does not bind directly to the LTR DNA, but complexes with cellular transcriptional regulator proteins that do so [there are similarities with polyomavirus (SV40, BK)

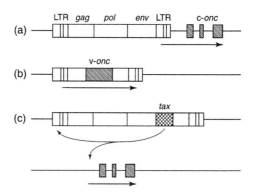

**Figure 1.1**. Models of oncogene activation by retroviruses. (a) Integration of a provirus adjacent to a cellular oncogene. The promoter region in the long terminal repeat (LTR) activates the oncogene. Note that enhancer regions in the LTR can also lead to upregula-tion of cellular oncogene activity, in which case the retrovirus may integrate either upstream or downstream from the oncogene (not shown). (b) The oncogene is incorpo-rated into the viral genome. (c) Transcriptional activation by *tax*. Reprinted from Seminars in Cancer Biology, Vol. 3, Issue 3, R.A. Weiss, Retroviruses and human cancer, pp. 321–328, 1992, by permission of the publisher, Academic Press Limited, London.

T-antigen complexing with RB and p53 here]. But Tax not only transactivates the viral LTR, but also activates several cellular genes (see Section 6.5.3). For example, expression of the interleukin(IL)-2 receptor alpha chain, CD25, is greatly increased in HTLV-I leukaemia cells, allowing autocrine proliferation as the same cells release IL-2. The X gene of HBV also has transactivating properties (see Section 2.6.1).

Thus, retroviral oncogenesis can occur by activating cellular oncogenes, or on rare occasions by actually hijacking them and incorporating them into the viral genome. Oncogenic herpesviruses, which have much larger genomes (approximately 150 genes) than retroviruses (3–10 genes), have exploited similar mechanisms to stimulate cell proliferation, and to overcome a switch to apoptosis early in the infectious cycle. As with retroviruses, herpesviruses cause tumours in many vertebrate species, from Lucké renal carcinoma in frogs, Marek's disease T-cell lymphoma in chickens, and lymphoma in primates. It is interesting to contrast the two oncogenic human herpesviruses, EBV, and KSHV (HHV-8). Whereas EBV transactivates several cellular genes that play a role in cell growth and survival, KSHV has pirated some of these genes to incorporate them into its own genome (*Table 1.4*). Interestingly, in the case of the anti-apoptotic *bcl-2* gene, EBV exploits both routes: it transactivates the cellular gene and also carries its own pirated version, *BHRF1*.

Thus, there are many ways in which the viral genome interacts with host DNA, and in which viral proteins interact with host proteins. But it is important to remember that carcinogenesis is a multistep process. Only in the case of a few oncogene-carrying retroviruses do tumours appear as an early consequence of infection.

## 1.7 Prospects for prevention and control

The greatest prospect for significantly reducing the human cancer burden is through immunization against infection by oncogenic viruses (see Chapter 7).

**Table 1.4.** Cellular growth and survival genes activated or pirated by human oncogenic herpesviruses

| EBV | Cellular gene | HHV-8 |
|---|---|---|
| EBNA2, EBNA-LP | *cyclin D2* | v-*cyclin* |
| LMP-1,[a] EBNA3b,[a] BHRF1[b] | *bcl-2* | v-*bcl-2* |
| gp340/220 | *IL-6* | v-*IL6* |
| EBNA2 | *IFN resistance* | v-*IRF* |

HHV-8 carries its own homologues of the indicated cellular genes whereas EBV activates the cellular genes using its own gene products as indicated. In the case of *bcl-2*, EBV both [a] transactivates and [b] carries its own homologue. See Sections 4.7.2, 5.7, 5.8 and 5.9.

An efficacious, safe vaccine against HBV exists, although it will take 40 years to see a significant reduction in liver cancer – the sixth most common cause of cancer death worldwide. Vaccines designed to prevent infection by EBV, based on the major viral glycoprotein that elicits neutralizing antibodies, are almost ready to begin field trials. Their efficacy will probably first be tested on preventing infectious mononucleosis in students, but the potential to prevent nasopharyngeal carcinoma (NPC) is appealing. NPC is the commonest cancer in parts of southern China, affecting a risk group that represents about 8% of mankind.

Vaccines against the papillomaviruses associated with cervical carcinoma, HPV-16 and HPV-18, are also being actively pursued. However, these are at an earlier stage of development, and in the absence of a suitable animal model it will be difficult to test their efficacy. Whole, killed virions, and recombinant envelope vaccines in vaccinia vectors both protect monkeys and rabbits from infection by HTLV-I. Given the will and a sufficient market – a big if – an HTLV-I vaccine should be feasible. Regrettably, despite a much greater effort, the prospects for an HIV vaccine are much more problematic, because lentiviruses such as HIV escape immune surveillance more easily than oncoviruses.

Besides preventative vaccines, the prospects for early screening and treatment are also promising. Although the cytologists who do it may not realize it, screening for dyskaryotic cells in cervical smears is a type of viral screening. The dyskaryotic bodies are really papillomavirus inclusions. With the introduction of genotyping for HPV, more accurate screening could be introduced. Cervical cancer causes as many or possibly more deaths worldwide than breast cancer, so better screening and vaccination could help to eliminate a major scourge of women. Moreover, there is the possibility that a so-called therapeutic vaccine might be effective, whereby immunization after exposure to HPV may still prevent progression to cancer, or at least stop re-infection. In China, programmes have been set up to detect incipient NPC through screening for raised blood IgA levels specific to EBV (see Section 4.8.8). This allows identification of individuals with an early, non-invasive stage of the tumour, at a time when it can be treated successfully by local radiotherapy or surgery.

While intensive research on the known oncogenic viruses and the development of vaccines is of prime importance, a search for novel tumour viruses is also worthwhile. HHV-8, which now looks like a causative virus for KS and primary effusion lymphoma (see Chapter 5), was discovered and reported only at the end of 1994. There may be more human viruses for the next generation of viral oncologists to discover, dissect molecularly, and immunize against.

Finally, there is the prospect that viruses may be harnessed to treat cancer as well as to prevent it in the first place. Virus-based therapies are discussed in Chapter 7. Some viruses, for example certain parvoviruses, will replicate only in proliferating cells and therefore might be used to kill cancer cells selectively. A genetically modified adenovirus has been engineered to possess a similar property, in particular to replicate and kill p53-negative cells. Because approximately 50% of human tumours of multiple types lack p53, this virus is ready to undergo clinical trial. Viruses such as the avian paramyxovirus Newcastle disease virus have been used in the past to 'xenogenize' tumours, that is to enhance natural immune responses to the tumour through the expression of viral antigens. Retroviruses and adenoviruses have been adapted to act as vehicles for gene therapy. These missiles can be 'armed' with different kinds of weapons to attack cancer cells, such as genes encoding cytokines or proteins that enhance immune recognition (immunotherapy), and genes encoding enzymes that convert prodrugs into cytotoxic agents in the locality of the tumour. 'Curing' tumour cells by re-introducing functional tumour suppressor genes is less likely to become a practical option. While cancer gene therapy research is attracting much interest, there is a long way to go before such treatments become routine. Nevertheless, we can look forward to an exciting time in tumour virology and gene therapy.

## Further reading

**Coffin, J.M., Hughes, S.M. and Varmus, H.E.** (eds) (1997) *Retroviruses.* Cold Spring Harbor Laboratory Press, New York.

**Fields, B.N., Knipe, D.M. and Howley, P.M.** (eds) (1996) *Virology.* Lippincott-Raven, Philadelphia.

**Minson, A., Neil, J. and McCrae, M.** (eds) (1994) *Viruses and Cancer.* Cambridge University Press, Cambridge.

**Tooze, J.** (1982) *DNA Tumour Viruses.* Cold Spring Harbor Laboratory Press, New York.

Chapter 2

# Viral hepatitis and primary liver cancer

## Tim J. Harrison

## 2.1 Introduction

The discovery of hepatitis B surface antigen (HBsAg) in the 1960s, and sub-sequent development of serological assays, confirmed the association of chronic viral hepatitis with the development of primary liver cancer. Cloning of the hepatitis B virus (HBV) genome in 1979 made available hybridization probes which detected integrated HBV DNA in the vast majority of tumours from HBsAg-positive patients. Animal viruses related to HBV, particularly woodchuck hepatitis virus (WHV), were also associated with the development of liver cancer in their native hosts.

At least three mechanisms of viral oncogenesis were considered for HBV:

(i) insertion of the HBV genome disrupts normal cellular gene expression;
(ii) HBV encodes a transforming protein;
(iii) chronic hepatitis and the ensuing cellular regeneration and cirrhosis leads
   to liver cancer in a non-specific manner.

Many groups of scientists searched for evidence of insertional mutagenesis by sequencing clones from genomic libraries containing HBV and flanking cellular DNA. No common sites of HBV integration were found. Integration of HBV DNA is not part of the replication process (see Section 2.3) and seems to occur as a 'virological dead-end' with insertion of fragments of the genome randomly into the chromosomes. Occasionally, HBV DNA has been found inserted in or adjacent to cellular genes where a change in expression may disrupt control of cell growth (see Section 2.5).

HBV and its DNA fail to transform cells in culture. The long delay between initial infection and development of cancer also argues against a direct mech-anism of transformation by a viral gene product. Nonetheless, the discovery

*Viruses and Human Cancer*, edited by J.R. Arrand and D.R. Harper
© 1998 BIOS Scientific Publishers Ltd, Oxford

that the *x*-gene product, so-called because its function originally was obscure, functions as a transcriptional transactivator, has led to interest in a possible role in oncogenesis (see Section 2.6).

The recent discovery of hepatitis C virus (HCV) and the recognition that chronic hepatitis C also may lead to liver cancer demands another perspective. HCV is an RNA virus, there is no DNA intermediate in its replication, nor can the genome integrate into cellular chromosomes. Presumably, HCV has a non-specific role, as outlined above, in the progression to tumour and this may be true, in some instances, for HBV also.

## 2.2 The epidemiological association of HBV infection with primary liver cancer

Hepatocellular carcinoma (HCC) is one of the 10 most common cancers in man with over 250 000 new cases worldwide each year. In areas where the tumour is particularly common, for example, some regions of sub-Saharan Africa, China and South-East Asia, the age-adjusted incidence of HCC is over 30 new cases per 100 000 population each year; whereas it is less than five cases per 100 000 per year in Western Europe and North America. Primary liver cancer is more common among males than females and the incidence of the tumour increases with age, reaching a peak in the 30–50 year age group. This age/sex distribution is similar to that observed for EBV-related naso-pharyngeal carcinoma (see Section 4.8.8).

Following the introduction of specific tests for the serological markers of HBV infection, it became clear that the geographical areas with a high inci-dence of primary liver cancer were coincident with those with a high preva-lence of seropositivity for HBsAg (*Figure 2.1*). Furthermore, most patients from high risk areas presenting with primary liver cancer proved to be HBsAg-positive or to have high titres of antibodies to the viral nucleoprotein (anti-HBc)[1,2]. HBV infection in these areas usually occurs at a young age, either following perinatal infection from a carrier mother or through horizontal trans-mission in early childhood. Thus, there is often a considerable interval between the initial virus infection and development of HCC, although tumours may occur in younger age groups in high risk populations.

The relative risk of an HBsAg-carrier, compared to a matched, non-carrier, developing primary liver cancer was estimated in an elegant prospective study performed in Taiwan by Beasley and co-workers [3]. Over 22 000 men, including more than 3 000 HBsAg carriers, were followed for 75 000 man-years. The HBsAg carriers proved more than 200-fold more likely to develop HCC than members of the non-carrier group and more than 50% of the deaths in the former group were due to the tumour or to cirrhosis, another possible consequence of long-term HBV infection [4]. However, HCC may develop in HBsAg-positive patients in the absence of underlying cirrhosis.

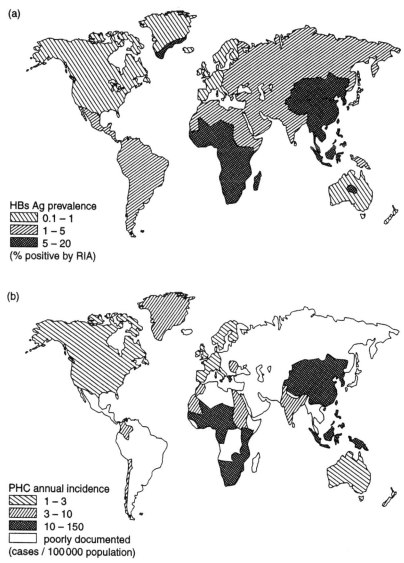

**Figure 2.1.** Prevalence of hepatitis B surface antigen (a) and incidence of primary liver cancer (b) worldwide. Redrawn with permission from S. Karger AG, Basel, from Maupas and Melnick, 1981, Progress in Medical Virology Vol. 27.

## 2.3 Replication of hepatitis B virus

### 2.3.1 The structure of the genome

The HBV virion is a 42 nm particle comprising a nucleocapsid enveloped by HBsAg embedded in lipid derived from the host cell. The 27 nm nucleocapsid is composed of HBV core antigen (HBcAg) surrounding the genome and at least one molecule of the virus-specified polymerase. The 3.2 kb genome has

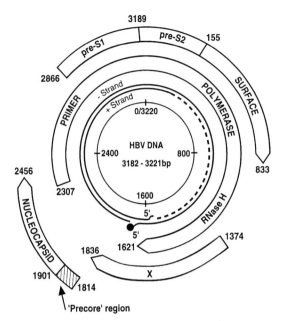

**Figure 2.2.** Structure and organization of the hepatitis B virus genome showing open reading frames and multiple start sites in the core and surface regions. Note the compact organization: all nucleotides encode protein and around half are located where reading frames overlap, all *cis*-acting elements are embedded within coding sequence. 3182–3221 bp refers to the extremes of observed genome size.

an unusual structure – the 5' ends of the two linear strands of DNA overlap in the cohesive end region of around 240 nt, maintaining a circular configuration (*Figure 2.2*). The minus strand, which has opposite polarity to all of the viral transcripts, has a terminal redundancy of nine nucleotides. The plus strand, however, is incomplete and up to 40% of the genome is single-stranded. The polymerase in the virion is able to complete plus strand synthesis *in vitro* if the virus coat is solubilized and dNTPs are provided. Primers for viral DNA synthesis remain covalently attached to both 5' ends in the virion. The minus strand primer is a protein which is linked to the DNA through a tyrosine residue and the plus strand primer is a capped oligoribonucleotide 18 bases in length.

### 2.3.2 The template for transcription

Following infection, the genome is converted to a covalently closed, circular (ccc) form which is located in the nucleus. Supercoiled HBV DNA is the template for transcription of all of the messenger RNAs and the pregenomic RNA, an intermediate in genome replication. The viral DNA does not integrate into chromosomal DNA during productive infection. The process of conversion of virion to ccc DNA is poorly understood but must involve completion of the plus strand, presumably by the endogenous polymerase, removal of the primers and ligation of the ends of the two strands. These early events may be crucial to the oncogenic process because data from the analysis of integrated HBV DNA suggest that it is virion DNA or intermediates in this conversion which recombine with cellular DNA during abortive infections.

During productive infection, the ccc DNA is transcribed from at least four promoters (*Figure 2.3*). All of the RNAs are 3' co-terminal and are polyadenylated in response to a signal in the core open reading frame (ORF). Transcripts from the core promoter are greater than genome length, around 3.5 kb. This promoter lacks a TATA box and the cap sites are heterogeneous. The pregenomic RNA, with 5' ends most distal from the promoter, is an intermediate in genome replication, as well as acting as message for HBcAg and the polymerase. The precore RNA, which has additional sequences at the 5' end, is translated into the precursor (p25) of the secreted protein, HBeAg. The pregenomic RNA is packaged with the polymerase in immature core particles in the cytoplasm. A stem–loop structure at the 5' end of the pregenome, the ε or packaging signal, is essential for this process.

### 2.3.3 Genome replication

The polymerase may be subdivided into four domains [5]. The amino-terminal domain acts as the primer for minus strand DNA synthesis and remains covalently attached to the 5'end of that strand in the mature virion. This is followed by a spacer region or tether, the DNA- and RNA-dependent DNA polymerase and, at the carboxyl terminus, an RNase H activity. There is no evidence of an integrase activity analogous to that in retroviral reverse transcriptases.

It is not clear whether the pregenome is packaged with two polymerase

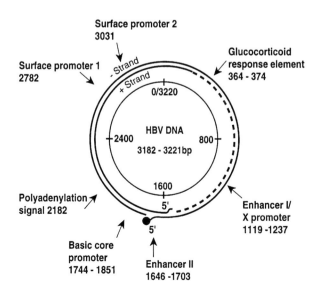

**Figure 2.3.** *Cis*-acting elements in the hepatitis B virus genome.

molecules which act as primer and polymerase or whether both functions are provided by one molecule. The latter alternative is attractive because the ensuing topological constraints may facilitate template switching by the polymerase during genome synthesis. Priming of DNA synthesis occurs at the position of the ε packaging signal with the synthesis of a nascent strand four nucleotides long [6]. The primer and nascent strand then seem to undergo a template switch to a complementary (τ) sequence near to the 3' end of the pregenome. Minus strand synthesis then proceeds by reverse transcription of the pregenome with concomitant degradation of the template (RNase H-like activity). The remaining capped oligoribonucleotide (which was the 5' end of the pregenome) is at the position of the direct repeat, DR1, and is now believed to translocate to the other copy of the direct repeat, DR2, on the minus strand and to prime synthesis of the plus strand. The short terminal redundancy of the minus strand permits circularization of the genome, with another template switch by the polymerase, as the plus strand is synthesized. Completion of the core presumably starves the polymerase of precursor nucleoside triphosphates leaving the plus strand incomplete. The cores are then coated with HBsAg to form mature virus particles. Early in infection, some nascent progeny genomes are recycled to the nucleus to build up the pool of ccc templates. It is possible that aberrant chromosomal integration of HBV DNA occurs during this process also.

### 2.3.4 Expression of viral proteins

As noted above, species of the 3.5 kb family of RNAs act as messengers for translation of hepatitis B core antigen (HBcAg), a secreted protein (HBeAg) and the polymerase. The core open reading frame (ORF) has two in-phase initiation codons (*Figure 2.2*). Messenger RNAs with 5' ends most distal from the promoter are translated from the second AUG to the 22 kDa HBcAg. The carboxyl terminus of this protein is extremely rich in basic residues, predominantly arginine, and may interact with viral nucleic acid. Messenger RNAs with more proximal 5' ends (precore RNA) are translated from the first AUG to a 25 kDa precursor protein (p25). The additional 29 residues at the amino terminus include a signal sequence which locates the protein in the endoplasmic reticulum where the first 19 amino acids are cleaved off by a cellular signal peptidase. The 17 kDa HBeAg is secreted following further processing by the Golgi apparatus including proteolytic removal of the basic, carboxyl-terminal domain. The polymerase seems to be translated from the pregenomic RNA, following internal initiation by ribosomes.

Northern blot analysis of HBV RNA in chronically infected livers reveals 3.5 and 2.1 kb species. The latter are transcribed from a promoter in the preS1 region and are mRNAs for HBsAg. This promoter resembles the SV40 late promoter, lacking a TATA box, and again, the cap sites are heterogeneous. The surface ORF has three in-phase initiation codons which are used to translate the various forms of HBsAg. Most of the 2.1 kb RNAs are translated from the downstream initiation codon to the 226 amino acid major surface protein, p24, which also may be glycosylated, gp27. Translation from the second AUG yields the two middle proteins, gp33 and gp36, with an additional 55 residues (preS2 domain) at the amino terminus. Messenger RNA for the large surface proteins, p39 and gp42 which include the preS1 domain, are rather less abundant and are transcribed from a second surface promoter further upstream (*Figure 2.3*). RNA transcribed from the fourth promoter is around 0.8 kb in size and is translated into the 154 amino acid X protein, which is now known to function as a transcriptional transactivator [7] and may up-regulate transcription from the core, and perhaps other, promoters during productive infection.

## 2.4 Integration of the HBV genome

### 2.4.1 Tumour cell lines

Primary liver tumours from HBsAg-positive patients frequently stain positive for HBsAg. The first successful attempt at the long-term culture of cells from such a tumour yielded a cell line (PLC/PRF/5) which secretes HBsAg into the medium [8]. Southern hybridization analysis of this line shows integration of HBV DNA at several sites (*Figure 2.4*, lane 1). Further analysis reveals considerable rearrangement of the viral DNA, although it is not clear whether these rearrangements were present in the original tumour or occurred during the establishment of the cell line. Confirmation of the integration of transcriptionally active HBV DNA in primary liver tumours gave strong support to the hypothesis of a direct viral role in the oncogenic process. The subsequent detection in PLC/PRF/5 cells of transcripts running from viral into cellular sequences [9] was consistent with a promoter insertion mechanism of oncogenesis.

Following the early success of Alexander and co-workers [8], others have been successful in establishing cell lines from primary liver tumours. Many contain integrated HBV DNA although by no means all of those express HBsAg.

### 2.4.2 Integration in tumour DNA

Many researchers have studied HBV DNA integration in HCC [10–13]. At least 80% of tumours from HBsAg-positive patients contain viral integrants which are detectable by hybridization (*Figure 2.4*, lane 5), although small integrants may have been missed in some cases. It is possible that more sensitive techniques, such as the polymerase chain reaction (PCR), may enable the detection of viral DNA sequences in tumours which appear negative by hybridization. Frequently, HBV DNA is integrated at multiple sites, indeed, tumours containing viral DNA integrated at a single site seem relatively uncommon. Furthermore, the patterns of integration observed suggested the

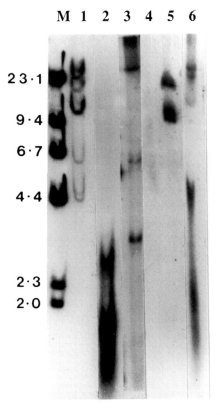

**Figure 2.4.** Composite illustrating the state of the HBV genome in liver determined by Southern hybridization. Lane 1, integration in the PLC/PRF/5 cell line; lane 2, replicative intermediates in the biopsy of an HBeAg-positive carrier; lane 3, integration in the biopsy of an anti-HBe-positive patient; lanes 4 and 5, non-tumorous and tumour tissue from an anti-HBe-positive carrier (partial hepatectomy); lane 6, biopsy from an HBeAg-positive carrier showing replicative forms and integrated HBV DNA. All DNA samples were digested with *Hind*III which does not cut HBV DNA. Lane M, molecular weight markers (λ/*Hin*d III), sizes in kb to the left. Modified from [20].

sites of integration in the human genome are random, although chromosomes 11 and 17 seem to be represented more than average [14]. Tumours usually are clonal with respect to HBV DNA integration, seemingly having arisen from a single cell following the integration event.

The structure of HBV integrants has been determined for a number of tumours, usually following selection and analysis of clones of HBV and flanking cellular DNA from genomic libraries. Compilation of the data from many such studies [15] reveals that the virus host junctions are not random with respect to the viral DNA. Integration frequently occurs around the 5' ends of the genomic strands in the region of the direct repeats. It has been suggested that the terminal redundancy of the minus strand may result in a triple-stranded structure which is a target for recombination. Integration interrupts one or more viral genes and integrants of greater than genome length and which might act as templates for the production of infectious virus have not been reported.

As noted above, the tumour cell line PLC/PRF/5 secretes HBsAg and synthesis of the surface protein by tumours is not uncommon. Hsu *et al.* [16] analysed 204 tumours from cases in Taiwan and found that around 32% expressed HBsAg. Thus, integrated DNA may be transcribed from the surface promoter(s) and, because a virus/host junction is likely to occur between the promoter and polyadenylation signal, these transcripts may run into cellular sequences. In some cases, the surface ORF will itself be interrupted, leading to the synthesis of surface proteins which are truncated or fused to domains specified by cellular sequences. Such truncated surface proteins may function as transactivators, as discussed below.

Expression of products of the core ORF in tumours, on the other hand, seems much less common (only 14.7% of tumours in the study cited above [16]). A number of factors may account for this. Firstly, integrants with virus/host junctions near to DR1 may not include the core promoter. Secondly, methylation of integrated HBV DNA [17] may affect expression of the core ORF. Thirdly, clones which express the core ORF from integrated DNA may be targeted for lysis by cytotoxic T cells and therefore not progress to tumours. The X promoter also may be active in viral integrants [18].

Intermediates of HBV replication are detected rarely in primary liver tumours. For example, Chen *et al.* [13,19] analysed patterns of integration of HBV DNA in 31 tumours from Taiwanese patients. In only four of these cases were replicative intermediates detected and this may have been attributable to contamination of the samples with non-tumorous tissue. If preneoplastic clones with integrated HBV DNA are resistant to superinfection they may have a selective advantage in a regenerating liver with chronic active hepatitis B. Although replicative and integrated HBV DNA may sometimes be observed in a particular biopsy (*Figure 2.4,* lane 6) it is not clear that both can occur in the same infected cell.

### 2.4.3 Integration in non-tumorous tissue

Integration of HBV DNA is not restricted to tumorous tissue. Analysis of liver biopsies from patients with chronic hepatitis B but without detectable tumours frequently reveals evidence of integration (*Figure 2.4,* lane 2) [11,20]. In fact, integration may occur as early as in the acute phase of infection. Detection of specific hybridization bands in non-tumorous tissue implies that integration has occurred at the same site(s) in many cells or that a single cell has expanded clonally following an integration event. There is no evidence for specific targets for integration of viral DNA in the human genome, and these data seem to indicate expansion of what may be pre-neoplastic clones.

Chronic hepatitis B is defined usually by the persistence of HBsAg in serum for more than 6 months. Acute HBV infection progresses to chronicity in only 5–10% of immunocompetent adults. Development of persistent infection is more common in the very young, particularly infants infected peri-natally from a carrier mother, who may develop persistent infections with rates as high as 90%. These high rates of progression to chronicity have been attrib-uted to the immaturity of the neonatal immune system and the tolerizing effects of maternal anti-HBc and HBeAg which may cross the placenta.

The chronic carrier state may be divided into two phases. In the first, HBV replicates actively in the hepatocytes and the individual is viraemic. This phase is usually associated with sero-positivity for HBeAg which is secreted from the infected hepatocytes. Over a period of months or years, levels of virus replication may decline with clearance of infected hepatocytes from the liver and eventual seroconversion from HBeAg- to anti-HBe positivity. Clearance of infected hepatocytes seems to be the result of targeting by cytotoxic T cells principally to products from the core ORF displayed on the cell surface. Antiviral therapy of patients with active virus replication, for example, using interferon or nucleoside analogues, seeks to hasten cessation of virus replica-tion and seroconversion to anti-HBe.

Not all viraemic individuals are seropositive for HBeAg. Synthesis of HBeAg is not an essential step in the virus replication cycle and infections with variants which are unable to synthesize this protein are not uncommon, partic-ularly in certain geographical regions such as the Mediterranean and Far East [21–23]. Many patients in these regions seem to be infected initially with a mixture of wild-type and variant virus and selection of the variant may occur during seroconversion to anti-HBe. Such variants usually have point muta-tions, often producing an in-phase termination codon, in the precore region of the genome. The detection in primary liver tumours of integrated HBV DNA with precore mutations has been reported but there is no evidence that these variants are any more tumorigenic than the wild-type virus.

The second phase of the carrier state is associated with continued surface antigenaemia in the absence of virus replication. In such individuals, synthesis of HBsAg may continue from hepatocytes with integrated viral genomes. Integration seems to occur throughout the replicative phase and cells and clones with integrated viral DNA may accumulate and expand clonally within the liver. A proportion of such clones may have the first of a series of genetic changes leading to neoplasia. This is consistent with the high rates of primary liver cancer in those who are infected at a young age and endure many years of active virus replication.

## 2.5 The search for evidence of *cis*-activation

Sequencing of the HBV genome almost 20 years ago did not provide evidence of a viral oncogene. Furthermore, attempts to transform cells *in vitro* with HBV DNA were unsuccessful and the long latency between HBV infection and development of HCC argued against the direct action of a viral gene product. Although we now know the X protein product and other proteins expressed from integrated HBV DNA may function as transactivators, there was formerly a great deal of enthusiasm for the hypothesis that the neoplastic process might be explained directly by insertional mutagenesis. In addition to the activity of the viral promoters other *cis*-acting sequences such as the enhancers and glucocorticoid-responsive element (*Figure 2.3*) may be present in viral integrants and cellular genes may be activated or inactivated directly by the insertional process and deletions [24] and translocations [25] which may ensue. The search for supportive data included analysis of integrants for evidence of proximity to cellular genes and the use of known oncogenes and proto-oncogenes to probe DNA and RNA extracted from tumours.

Such studies did not provide evidence of the frequent activation or inactivation of cellular genes. As noted above, there is no commonality among the integration sites in different tumours. HBV DNA is integrated frequently into *Alu* or other repetitive sequences, probably reflecting the size of such targets in the human genome.

### 2.5.1 A novel retinoic acid receptor

Dejean *et al.* [26] analysed the genomic sequences flanking a single viral integrant in a tumorous nodule and used these sequences, in turn, to identify the unoccupied site in non-tumorous liver. They reported integration of HBV DNA into sequences homologous to the oncogene v-*erbA* and steroid receptor genes and which later were identified as a novel retinoic acid receptor gene [27]. Retinoic acid is an important morphogen during embryogenesis and it is conceivable that a change in the receptor might contribute to the neoplastic process. However, a report of the up-regulation of the corresponding mRNA in other HCCs and tumour cell lines [28] has not been confirmed by others.

### 2.5.2 HBV integration in a cyclin A gene

Analysis of another single HBV DNA integrant in an early stage HCC revealed that the target site was an intron in a cyclin A gene [29]. Cyclins play a crucial role in the control of cell division and, in this isolated case, disruption of normal gene expression may have resulted in a loss of growth control.

It is possible that analysis of other tumours will identify further individual examples of altered expression of cellular genes following HBV DNA integration. However, most studies of this type have not been so rewarding and it is extremely unlikely that a cellular gene, the expression of which is directly influenced by HBV DNA integration in a significant proportion of HCC, has escaped detection. This contrasts sharply with the findings from the most extensively studied animal model of HBV-associated hepatocellular carcinoma.

### 2.5.3 The woodchuck model

HBV is now recognized as the prototype of a group of viruses (hepadnaviruses) which infect mammals and birds. WHV has approximately 70% nucleotide homology with HBV and shares all of the major features of genome organization and expression. WHV causes persistent infections in its natural host, the eastern woodchuck (*Marmotta monax*), with a high rate of progression to chronic liver disease and HCC. WHV-infected woodchucks have been used extensively as a model for human HCC (reviewed by Buendia [30]).

Briefly, WHV DNA in tumours is often found to be integrated in or near to *myc* genes and is implicated in increased levels of *myc* RNA. Initial observations implicated the c-*myc* gene [31,32] but N-*myc* genes are involved more frequently [33,34]. In fact, the woodchuck genome has an extra copy of N-*myc*, termed N-*myc2*, which has the characteristics of a retrotransposed pseudogene, including an absence of introns. N-*myc2* is by far the most common target for WHV DNA integration in tumours, accounting for around 25% of the integration events which have been analysed [30]. Activation of *myc* genes may promote cell proliferation and this seems to be a key step in liver carcinogenesis in this model.

There is no equivalent of N-*myc2* in the human genome and direct activation of *myc* genes by HBV has not been reported in human HCCs. The relevance of this model to human liver cancer is, therefore, questionable.

## 2.6 Transactivation by viral gene products

Failure to find evidence of *cis*-activation in the majority of HBV-associated tumours prompted a reconsideration of the possible role of HBV gene products. In particular, the X protein was shown to function as a transcriptional transactivator [7], consistent with a role in the oncogenic process. Furthermore, patients with HCC were frequently found to be seropositive for antibodies which reacted with recombinant *x* gene products [35] or synthetic peptides derived from the predicted amino acid sequence [36]. Levels of X protein in primary liver tumours seem to be rather higher than in chronically infected liver tissue but it is not clear how *HBx* gene expression may be upregulated.

### 2.6.1 Transactivation by the X gene product

Transactivation has been studied *in vitro* by co-transfecting cells with plasmids which express the *x* gene product and reporter genes such as for chloramphenicol acetyl transferase (CAT) and firefly luciferase under the control of a variety of promoter and enhancer sequences. All four promoters in the HBV genome, including the X promoter, are upregulated by the *x* gene product [37]. The X and core promoters are associated with enhancers, (EnI and EnII, respectively, *Figure 2.3*) and it has proved difficult to dissect the effects of X on the individual elements.

The role of the *x* gene product *in vivo* remains unclear although it seems likely that it acts early in the replicative cycle, upregulating viral transcription.

Studies with the woodchuck virus suggest the WHV *x* gene homologue is required by that hepadnavirus for the establishment of infection [38]. However, that HBV genomes without functional X ORFs seem viable in that hepatitis B virions may be expressed in cells in culture from HBV DNA with codon 8 of the *HBx* ORF modified to a termination codon (without disrupting the polymerase) [39]. Avian hepadnaviruses do not have a homologue of the X ORF and it may have been transduced from the host genome during the evolution of the mammalian viruses. Consistent with this hypothesis is the observation that codon usage in the X ORF resembles that of eukaryotic cellular genes more than that of eukaryotic viruses.

The *x* gene product also can transactivate the promoters of other viruses, including the early promoters of SV40 and adenoviruses and the long terminal repeats (LTRs) of human immune deficiency virus and other retroviruses [37]. A variety of mammalian promoters also are effective targets of transactivation, including those of β-interferon and c-*myc* genes [40]. However, the *x* gene product does not bind directly to DNA. Transactivation by the X protein seems to be through responsive elements such as the transcription factor AP-1 (*jun–fos*) [41], AP-2 [42], NF-κB [43] and CRE [44] sites.

One mechanism of transactivation by the X protein seems dependent upon an Ap-1 binding site; a minimal promoter comprising a TATA box and an Sp1 site was not activated but inclusion of a tandem array of three AP-1 binding sites upstream resulted in a greater than five-fold increase in CAT activity [45]. X Protein activation of the AP-1-dependent promoter requires Ha-Ras and Raf-1 since expression of dominant-negative mutants block this effect [45,46]. In summary, the *x* gene product seems to act upstream of *ras/raf* in the activation pathway [47], although it is not clear that it interacts directly with either protein. Indeed, evidence that the X protein also may activate transcription through *ras/raf*-independent pathways argues that it may act rather further upstream in the signalling cascade.

The above observations are consistent with a role for the X protein in the oncogenic process. It should be noted, however, that the downstream half of the X ORF overlaps the direct repeats and thus may be disrupted frequently during integration. Furthermore, domain(s) in the carboxyl-terminus portion of the protein seem to be essential for transactivation and relatively few residues can be deleted from the carboxyl-terminus before activity is lost. In some cases, fusions of the X transactivating domain and host-encoded polypeptide sequences may be functional. Other data suggest a domain in the N-terminal portion of the X protein has a regulatory function and expression of this region alone may lead to *trans*-repression of *HBx* transactivation [48].

As noted above, initial attempts to transform susceptible cells in culture with HBV or HBV DNA were unsuccessful. More recently, Shirakata *et al.* [49] reported growth stimulation and tumorigenic transformation of NIH 3T3 cells by the *HBx* gene. Other studies [50] suggest that *HBx* may be sufficient to transform immortalized cell lines to the ability to grow in soft agar and induce tumours in nude mice. Reports of the effect of *HBx* as a transgene are contradictory. Transgenic mice in which the *x* gene was under the control of the α-1-antitrypsin regulatory region alone did not develop serious liver damage or HCC but levels of expression of the X protein were variable [51]. Transgenics with the *HBx* gene under the control of its own regulatory elements developed multifocal areas of altered hepatocytes progressing to benign adenomas and then malignant carcinomas [52].

The X protein recently has been shown to interact with a cellular protein (XAP-1) which is involved in nucleotide excision repair of damaged DNA [52a]. Expression of HBx *in vitro* significantly inhibited the ability of cells to repair damaged DNA. Clearly, long term expression of HBx may play a role in hepatocarcinogenesis if DNA repair is inhibited *in vivo*.

### 2.6.2 Other viral transactivators

An investigation of the transactiviating potential of a single 5.6 kb integrant in the HCC cell line HuH-4, comprising rearranged HBV DNA including the *HBx* gene, led to a surprising discovery [53]. In addition to a subclone containing the entire X ORF, two further subclones without *HBx* sequences were found to transactivate a CAT gene driven by the SV40 early promoter. These subclones were found to express a pre-S2 protein which was C-terminally truncated by a virus/host junction. Artificially constructed plasmids expressing pre-S2/S truncations also were found to have a similar effect. An HCC with a single integrant of HBV DNA again produced a truncated pre-S/S protein with a transactivator function. Truncated pre-S/S proteins may bind to protein kinase C and activate AP-1-dependent promoters through a Raf-1 dependent pathway [54].

A recent report of the transactivating potential of a fragment of the major surface protein [55] awaits confirmation. In this study, the authors used multiple, overlapping PCR to identify a region of the surface ORF integrated in 22 out of 36 HCC tissue samples. They went on to show an approximately three-fold increase in the activity of a luciferase reporter driven by the HBV EnI/X promoter complex when cotransfected with plasmids expressing fragments of the major surface protein.

## 2.7 Other factors

Development of human cancer is widely regarded to be multifactorial (see also Sections 1.3, 3.6 and 4.9) and to involve several (mutagenic) hits. In addition to HBV, dietary factors, smoking, other hepatotropic viruses and other factors may have a causal role in the development of HCC.

### 2.7.1 Dietary factors

In some areas of the world with a high incidence of HCC, contamination of foodstuffs with mycotoxins such as aflatoxin is not uncommon. Aflatoxin is known to cause HCC when fed experimentally to rats and its possible role in human HCC, for example in causing p53 mutations (see below), is unclear. In some areas of mainland China, the incidence of HCC varies widely on a background of high prevalence of HBsAg and this may be explained by carcinogens in the diet. By careful control of diet, it has been possible to demonstrate that WHV infection is sufficient to produce tumours in woodchucks in the absence of dietary co-factors [56]. However, as noted above, the extremely high incidence of WHV-associated HCC in woodchucks casts doubt on the applicability of this model to the situation in man.

### 2.7.2 The role of p53

Mutations in the *p53* tumour suppressor gene are the most commonly detected genetic alterations in human malignancies. *p53* mutations have been observed in HCCs from high risk areas such as China and southern Africa [57]. In particular, a G to T transversion in codon 249 of the *p53* gene has commonly been observed and it has been suggested that exposure to aflatoxin may be associated with the mutation. Codon 249 mutations seem to be uncommon in HCC from areas with a low incidence of primary liver cancer, even in HBV-associated tumours. Some studies report that overexpression of p53 in primary liver tumours, particularly from low incidence areas, is not necessarily associated with mutations in the *p53* gene.

It is not clear whether there is any association between HBV and *p53*. It has been reported that the *x* gene product interacts directly with *p53* [58] but the insolubility of the X protein and its tendency to aggregate *in vitro* suggest that non-specific binding to other proteins may occur. There is at least one report of integration of HBV DNA near to the *p53* gene in chromosome 17p but it is not clear that the integration events had a direct effect on the gene [59]. Chronic expression of the X protein, in the context of wild-type *p53*, prompts cells to *p53*-mediated apoptosis [60] but this may not occur with *p53* gene mutations or conformational inactivation of *p53*.

### 2.7.3 The role of hepatitis C virus

For many years it was speculated that there was an association between at least one form of non-A, non-B hepatitis and development of HCC. In Japan, for example, the incidence of HCC has risen over the past 20 years despite a steady decrease in the prevalence of HBsAg. The discovery of HCV and the development of assays for anti-HCV antibodies confirmed its association with HCC.

Rates of anti-HCV positivity as high as 60–80% have been reported in HCC patients from areas of the world such as Italy, Spain and Japan where HBV infection is relatively uncommon. In areas such as Taiwan, where most HCC is HBV-associated, rates of anti-HCV are lower in HCC patients

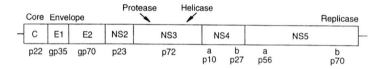

**Figure 2.5.** Genetic organization of the HCV genome. The 5' non-translated region contains *cis*-acting sequences believed to prime genome replication and an internal ribosome entry site (IRES) for translation of a large polyprotein. The carboxyl-terminal regions of the core and envelope proteins contain signal sequences and are cleaved in the endoplasmic reticulum by the cellular signal peptidase. Alternative cleavage sites at the carboxyl-terminus of E2 yield a theoretical 7 kDa protein, termed tp7 [62]. The NS2/NS3 junction is cleaved in *cis* by a metalloproteinase activity [63]. The remaining cleavages are carried out by the NS3 chymotrypsin-like protease, which requires NS4a as a co-factor [64]. Unlike the flaviviruses, NS5 is cleaved to NS5a and NS5b. NS5b contains the GDD motif common to RNA-dependent RNA polymerases and NS5a also may be involved in RNA replication. Helicase and ATPase activity in the carboxyl-terminal domain of NS3 are believed to be involved in unwinding the double-stranded RNA intermediate. The function of NS4b is not known. The original HCV isolate was believed to have polyA at the 3' end, and other isolates polyU, but further sequences at the 3' end may form a hairpin structure to prime RNA replication [65].

generally but high in the HBsAg-negative subset. Because acute, post-transfusion hepatitis was documented in many patients, it has been possible to determine that 20 or 30 years of chronic HCV infection precede the development of HCC. The association of HCV and HCC is reviewed extensively by Kiyosawa and Furuta [61].

HCV is a positive-sense RNA virus (*Figure 2.5*) related to the flaviviruses and (more closely to) the pestiviruses and has been designated the prototype of a new genus of the *Flaviviridae*. By analogy with these related viruses, it would be expected that HCV replicates in the cytoplasm via generation of negative-sense RNA and partially double-stranded replicative intermediates and there is no evidence to the contrary. Thus, no DNA copy of the HCV genome is generated and viral nucleic acid does not integrate into chromosomal DNA. However, NIH3T3 cells transfected with cDNA clones expressing the region of the HCV genome designated NS3 had a transformed phenotype, including the ability to grow in soft agar [66]. More specifically, transformation was achieved with the 5' portion of NS3 which encodes a protease which may have cleaved and activated cellular proteins.

HCC seems to develop on a background of cirrhosis caused by long-term chronic active hepatitis and may be preceded by adenomatous hyperplastic nodules. There have been occasional reports of HCC developing in HCV-infected patients in the absence of underlying cirrhosis [67]. HCV isolates show a high degree of genetic diversity and have been classified phylogenetically into up to 10 major genotypes and a plethora of subtypes [68]. Whether some genotypes are more pathogenic and less responsive to treatment with interferon alpha remains controversial. Bruno *et al.* [69] and others have reported an increased risk of developing HCC for cirrhotic patients infected with genotype 1b, but an older age and increased duration of infection with this genotype, compared with other genotypes, may be a confounding factor. An increased frequency of HCC has been described in patients coinfected with HCV and human T-cell leukaemia virus type I (see Section 6.3.1.1).

### 2.7.4 An indirect role for HBV?

The findings with HCV invite a reappraisal of the role of HBV. Many have long argued that HBV causes HCC simply through the process of chronic active hepatitis, liver regeneration and cirrhosis. However, this hypothesis of a less direct role does not explain the finding of integrated HBV DNA in more than 80% of HBV-associated tumours. Furthermore, although HCC frequently develops on a background of cirrhosis, it is clear that tumours may also develop in HBV-infected livers without an intermediate cirrhotic stage (see also Section 1.5).

A further clue to the pathogenesis of HBV lies in a transgenic mouse model developed by Chisari and co-workers [70]. A motif in the pre-S1 domain of the large surface proteins directs virion assembly. Expression of the middle (pre-S2) and major surface proteins in cell culture results in their secretion but pre-S1 proteins are retained in the cytoplasm and inhibit the secretion of the other forms. Transgenic mice which express pre-S1 accumulate HBsAg in their livers resulting in the so-called ground glass hepatocytes, with hyper-plastic endoplasmic reticulum containing filamentous HBsAg particles, that are seen frequently in infected patients. These mice develop severe, prolonged hepatocellular injury with an inflammatory response, regenerative hyperplasia and, eventually, HCC.

## 2.8 Prognosis and treatment

Early detection is the key to successful treatment of primary liver cancer, the prognosis for treatment of symptomatic (late stage) cases is extremely poor. Many HCCs secrete alpha-fetoprotein (AFP) and serum levels are a valuable diagnostic marker. However, AFP levels may be insufficient for diagnosis until the tumour is beyond the treatable stage. Similarly, detection of tumours less than 1 cm in diameter using ultrasonography may be problematic. More sophisticated imaging techniques such as computerized tomography and magnetic resonance imaging are available but are not suitable for mass screening programmes. A combination of AFP measurement and ultrasonography may present the best compromise.

Five-year survival rates of greater than 40% have been achieved in several centres for surgical resection of small (less than 3–5 cm in diameter), single, well-differentiated (especially, encapsulated) tumours which have not been invaded by the hepatic vasculature. In cases where a tumour has developed in a cirrhotic liver, clearly the remaining liver will be diseased with a risk of development of further tumours and death from end-stage disease.

Liver transplantation is an alternative, especially for the cirrhotic patient. If the patient is viraemic, reinfection of the graft is almost inevitable. In the case of HBV, rapid progression to fibrosing cholestatic hepatitis has been reported [71]. Reinfection of older patients with HCV may be less of a problem because of the relatively slower progress of HCV disease.

Systemic chemotherapy is not usually an effective treatment for primary liver tumours and local, inter-arterial approaches are being investigated. Direct, percutaneous injection of sterile ethanol into small tumours has been used with some success and treatment of multiple tumours is possible using this approach. Transcatheter arterial embolization, for example with Gelfoam, induces necrosis of the tumour and may be used in combination with local chemotherapy.

## 2.9 Concluding remarks

Chronic infections with HBV and HCV viruses are associated with long-term liver damage, cirrhosis and the development of primary liver cancer. Both viruses seem to cause HCC through an indirect process involving liver regeneration, cirrhosis and the development of hyperplastic nodules. In addition, HBV is associated with the development of HCC in the absence of cirrhosis and the detection of integrated viral DNA in more than 80% of tumours from HBsAg-positive patients suggests a more direct role.

Transactivation of cellular transcription by HBV gene products may contribute to tumorigenesis but the long latent period to tumour development implies that other factors are involved. Activation or inactivation of cellular genes in *cis* through integration of the viral genome may play a very minor role – few examples have emerged following extensive studies in many laboratories. It is possible that further mechanisms whereby HBV contributes to hepatic carcinogenesis will be described in the future but it seems unlikely that a mechanism which applies to a large percentage of tumours has escaped notice.

Safe and effective vaccines are now available for the prevention of HBV infection (see Chapter 7). Mass immunization programmes are already underway and the World Health Organisation recommends worldwide universal infant immunization. In the years to come, we will see whether these programmes result in a significant reduction in the incidence of primary liver cancer. The immediate prospects for a hepatitis C vaccine, however, look rather bleak (see Section 7.3).

## References

1. **Maupas, P. and Melnick, J.L.** (1981) *Prog. Med. Virol.* **27:** 1–5.
2. **Szmuness, W.** (1978) *Prog. Med. Virol.* **24:** 40–69.

3. **Beasley, R.P., Hwang, L.Y., Lin, C.C. and Chien, C.S.** (1981) *Lancet* **2**:1129–113 3.
4. **Beasley, R.P. and Hwang, L.-Y.** (1991) in *Viral Hepatitis and Liver Disease.* (eds F.B. Hollinger, S.M. Lemon and H.S. Margolis). Williams and Wilkins, Baltimore: p. 532.
5. **Radziwill, G., Tucker W. and Schaller, H.** (1990) *J. Virol.* **64**: 613–620.
6. **Wang, G.-H. and Seeger, C.** (1993) *J. Virol.* **67**: 6507–6512.
7. **Twu, J.S. and Schloemer, R.H.** (1987) *J. Virol.* **61**: 3448–3453.
8. **MacNab, G.M., Alexander, J.J., Lecatsas, G., Bey, E.M. and Urbanowicz, J.M.** (1976) *Br. J. Cancer* **34**: 509–515.
9. **von Loringhoven, A.F., Koch, S., Hofschneider, P.H. and Koshy, R.** (1985) *EMBO J.* **4**: 249–255.
10. **Brechot, C., Pourcel, C., Louise, A., Rain, B. and Tiollais, P.** (1980) *Nature* **286**: 533–535.
11. **Shafritz, D.A., Shouval, D., Sherman, H.I., Hadziyannis, S.J. and Kew, M.C.** (1981) *N. Engl. J. Med.* **305**: 1067–1073.
12. **Hino, O., Kitagawa, T., Koike, K., Kobayashi, M., Hara, M., Mori, W., Nakashima, T., Hattori, N. and Sugano, H.** (1984) *Hepatology* **4**: 90–95.
13. **Chen, J.Y., Harrison, T.J., Lee, C.S., Chen, D.S. and Zuckerman, A.J.** (1986) *Br. J. Exp. Pathol.* **67**: 279–288.
14. **Tokino, T. and Matsubara, K.** (1991) *J. Virol.* **65**: 6761–6764.
15. **Nagaya, T., Nakamura, T., Tokino, T., Tsurimoto, T., Imai, M., Mayumi, T., Kamino, K., Yamamura, K. and Matsubara, K.** (1987) *Genes Dev.* **1**: 773–782.
16. **Hsu, H.C., Wu, T.T., Sheu, J.C., Wu, C.Y., Chiou, T.J., Lee, C.S. and Chen, D.S.** (1989) *Hepatology* **9**: 747–750.
17. **Chen, J.Y., Hsu, H.C., Lee, C.S., Chen, D.S., Zuckerman, A.J. and Harrison, T.J.** (1988) *J. Virol. Methods* **19**: 257–263.
18. **Diamantis, I.D., McGandy, C.E., Chen, T.J., Liaw, Y.F., Gudat, F. and Bianchi, L.** (1992) *J. Hepatol* **15**: 400–403.
19. **Chen, J.Y., Harrison, T.J., Lee, C.S., Chen, D.S. and Zuckerman, A.J.** (1988) *Hepatology* **8**: 518–523.
20. **Harrison, T.J., Anderson, M.G., Murray-Lyon, I.M. and Zuckerman, A.J.** (1986) *J. Hepatol.* **2**: 1–10.
21. **Carman, W.F., Jacyna, M.R., Hadziyannis, S., Karayiannis, P., McGarvey, M.J., Makris, A. and Thomas, H.C.** (1989) *Lancet* **2**: 588–591.
22. **Brunetto, M.R., Stemler, M., Bonino, F., Schodel, F., Oliveri, F., Rizzetto, M.,Verme, G. and Will, H.** (1990) *J. Hepatol.* **10**: 258–261.
23. **Carman, W.F., Ferrao, M., Lok, A.S., Ma, O.C., Lai, C.L. and Thomas, H.C.** (1992) *J. Infect. Dis.* **165**: 127–133.
24. **Rogler, C.E., Sherman, M., Su, C.Y., Shafritz, D.A., Summers, J., Shows, T.B. and Kew, M.** (1985) *Science* **230**: 319–322.
25. **Hino, O., Shows, T.B. and Rogler, C.E.** (1986) *Proc. Natl. Acad. Sci. USA* **83**: 8338–8342.
26. **Dejean, A., Bougueleret, L., Grzeschik, K.H. and Tiollais, P.** (1986) *Nature* **322**: 70–72.
27. **Brand, N., Petkovich, M., Krust, A., Chambon, P., de The, H., Marchio, A., Tiollais, P. and Dejean, A.** (1988) *Nature* **332**: 850–853.
28. **de Thé, H., Marchio, A., Tiollais, P. and Dejean, A.** (1987) *Nature* **330**: 667–670.
29. **Wang, J., Chenivesse, X., Henglein, B. and Brechot, C.** (1990) *Nature* **343**: 555–557.

30. **Buendia, M.A.** (1994) in *Viruses and Cancer.* (eds A. Minson, J. Neil and M. McCrae). Cambridge University Press, Cambridge, pp. 173–187.
31. **Moroy, T., Marchio, A., Etiemble, J., Trepo, C., Tiollais, P and Buendia, M.A.** (1986) *Nature* **324**: 276–279.
32. **Hsu, T., Moroy, T., Etiemble, J., Louise, A., Trepo, C., Tiollais, P. and Buendia, M.A.** (1988) *Cell* **55**: 627–635.
33. **Fourel, G., Trepo, C., Bougueleret, L., Henglein, B., Ponzetto, A., Tiollais, P. and Buendia, M.A.** (1990) *Nature* **347**: 294–298.
34. **Hansen, L.J., Tennant, B.C., Seeger, C. and Ganem, D.** (1993) *Mol. Cell Biol.* **13**: 659–667.
35. **Kay, A., Mandart, E., Trepo, C. and Galibert, F.** (1985) *EMBO J.* **4**: 1287–1292.
36. **Moriarty, A.M., Alexander, H., Lerner, R.A. and Thornton, G.B.** (1985) *Science* **227**: 429–433.
37. **Rossner, M.T.** (1992) *J. Med. Virol.* **36**: 101–117.
38. **Zoulim, F., Saputelli, J. and Seeger, C.** (1994) *J. Virol.* **68**: 2026–2030.
39. **Blum, H.E., Zhang, Z.S., Galun, E., Vonweizsacker, F., Garner, B., Liang, T.J. and Wands, J.R.** (1992) *J. Virol.* **66**: 1223–1227.
40. **Zhou, D.X. and Yen, T.S.** (1990) *J. Biol. Chem.* **265**: 20731–20734.
41. **Kekule, A.S., Lauer, U., Weiss, L., Luber, B. and Hofschneider, P.H.** (1993) *Nature* **361**: 742–745.
42. **Seto, E., Mitchell, P.J. and Yen, T.S.** (1990) *Nature* **344**: 72–74.
43. **Lucito, R. and Schneider, R.J.** (1992) *J. Virol.* **66**: 983–991.
44. **Williams, J.S. and Andrisani, O.M.** (1995) *Proc. Natl. Acad. Sci. USA* **92**: 3819–3823.
45. **Cross, J.C., Wen, P. and Rutter, W.J.** (1993) *Proc. Natl. Acad. Sci. USA* **90**: 8078–8082.
46. **Natoli, G., Avantaggiati, M.L., Chirillo, P., Puri, P., Ianni, A., Balsano, C. and Levrero, M.** (1994) *Oncogene* **9**: 2837–2843.
47. **Benn, J. and Schneider, R.J.** (1994) *Proc. Natl. Acad. Sci. USA* **91**: 10350–10354.
48. **Murakami, S., Cheong, J.H. and Kaneko, S.** (1994) *J. Biol. Chem.* **269**: 15118–15123.
49. **Shirakata, Y., Kawada, M., Fujiki, Y., Sano, H., Oda, M., Yaginuma, K., Kobayashi, M. and Koike, K.** (1989) *Jpn. J. Cancer Res.* **80**: 617–621.
50. **Hohne, M., Schaefer, S., Seifer, M., Feitelson, M.A., Paul, D. and Gerlich, W.H.** (1990) *EMBO J.* **9**: 1137–1145.
51. **Lee, T.H., Finegold, M.J., Shen, R.F., DeMayo, J.L., Woo, S.L. and Butel, J.S.** (1990) *J. Virol.* **64**: 5939–5947.
52. **Kim, C.M., Koike, K., Saito, I., Miyamura, T. and Jay, G.** (1991) *Nature* **351**: 317–320.
52a. **Becker, S.A., Lee, T.H., Butel, J.S. and Slagel, B.L.** (1998) *J. Virol.* **72**: 266–272.
53. **Kekule, A.S., Lauer, U., Meyer, M., Caselmann, W.H., Hofschneider, P.H. and Koshy, R.** (1990) *Nature* **343**: 457–461.
54. **Meyer, M., Caselmann, W.H., Schluter, V., Schreck, R., Hofschneider, P.H. and Baeuerle, P.A.** (1992) *EMBO J.* **11**: 2991–3001.
55. **Ramesh, R., Panda, S.K., Jameel, S. and Rajasambandam, P.** (1994) *J. Gen. Virol.* **75**: 327–334.

56. Popper, H., Roth, L., Purcell, R.H., Tennant, B.C. and Gerin, J.L. (1987) *Proc. Natl. Acad. Sci. USA* **84**: 866–870.
57. Tabor, E. (1994) *J. Med. Virol.* **42**: 357–365.
58. Wang, X.W., Forrester, K., Yeh, H., Feitelson, M.A., Gu, J.R. and Harris, C.C. (1994) *Proc. Natl. Acad. Sci. USA* **91**: 2230–2234.
59. Slagle, B.L., Zhou, Y.Z. and Butel, J.S. (1991) *Cancer Res.* **51**: 49–54.
60. Chirillo, P., Pagano, S., Natoli, G., Puri, P.L., Burgio, V.L., Balsano, C. and Levrero, M. (1997) *Proc. Natl. Acad. Sci. USA* **94**: 8162–8167.
61. Kiyosawa, K. and Furuta, S. (1994) *Curr. Stud. Hematol. Blood Transfus.* **61**: 98–120.
62. Lin, C., Lindenbach, B.D., Pragai, B.M., McCourt, D.W. and Rice, C.M. (1994). *J. Virol.* **68**: 5063–5073.
63. Hijikata, M., Mizushima, H., Akagi, T., Mori, S., Kakiuchi, N., Kato, N., Tanaka, T., Kimura, K. and Shimotohno, K. (1993). *J. Virol.* **67**: 4665–4675.
64. Failla, C., Tomei, L. and Defrancesco, R. (1994). *J. Virol.* **68**: 3753–3760.
65. Tanaka, T., Kato, N., Cho, M.J., Sugiyama, K. and Shimotohno, K. (1996) *J. Virol.* **70**: 3307–3312.
66. Sakamuro, D., Furukawa T. and Takegami T. (1995) *J. Virol.* **69**: 3893–3896.
67. el-Rafaie, A., Savage, K., Bhattacharya, S., Khakoo, S., Harrison, T.J., el-Batanony, M., Soliman el-Nasr, S., Mokhtar, N., Scheuer, P.J. and Dhillon, A.P. (1996) *Hepatology* **24**: 277–285.
68. Simmonds, P., Alberti, A., Alter, H.J. *et al.* (1994) *Hepatology* **19**: 1321–1324.
69. Bruno, S., Silini E., Crosignani A., *et al.* (1997) *Hepatology* **25**: 754–758.
70. Chisari, F.V., Klopchin, K., Moriyama, T., Pasquinelli, C., Dunsford, H.A., Sell, S., Pinkert, C.A., Brinster, R.L. and Palmiter, R.D. (1989) *Cell* **59**: 1145–1156.
71. Perrillo, R.P. and Mason, A.L. (1993) *N. Engl. J. Med.* **329**: 1885–1887.

# Further Reading

Beasley, R.P. and Hwang, L.-Y. (1991) Overview on the epidemiology of hepatocellular carcinoma. in *Viral Hepatitis and Liver Disease*, (eds F. B. Hollinger, S.M. Lemon, and H. S. Margolis). Williams and Wilkins, Baltimore, pp.18.

Buendia, M.A. (1994) Hepatitis B viruses and liver cancer: the woodchuck model. in *Viruses and Cancer*, (eds A. Minson, J. Neil and M. McCrae). Cambridge University Press, Cambridge, pp.27–28.

Dusheiko, G.M., Hobbs, K.E., Dick, R., Burroughs, A.K. (1992) Treatment of small hepatocellular carcinomas. *Lancet*, **340**: 34–35.

Okuda, K. (1993) New trends in hepatocellular carcinoma [editorial]. *Int. J. Clin. Lab. Res.* **23**: 173.

Robinson, W.S. (1992) The role of hepatitis B virus in the development of primary hepatocellular carcinoma : Part I: *J. Gastroenterol. Hepatol.* **7**: 622; Part II: *J. Gastroenterol. Hepatol.*, **8**: 95.

**Rossner, M.T.** (1992) Hepatitis B virus X gene product - a promiscuous transcriptional activator. *J. Med. Virol.* **36:** 28–30.

**Schirmacher, P., Rogler, C.E and, Dienes, H.P.** (1993) Current pathogenetic and molecular concepts in viral liver carcinogenesis. *Virchows Archiv B-Cell Pathol. Incl. Mol. Pathol.* **63**: 71.

**Yen, T.S.B.** (1996) Hepadnaviral X protein: Review of recent progress. *J. Biomed. Sci.* **3:** 28–30.

Chapter 3

# Human papillomaviruses and cancer

## Andrew C. Phillips and Karen H. Vousden

## 3.1 Introduction

Papillomaviruses are small, epitheliotropic DNA viruses found in a wide variety of species. The human papillomavirus (HPV) group consists currently of more than 70 distinct types, causing lesions of the genital, upper respiratory and digestive tracts and cutaneous lesions at a variety of sites. Although there are diverse sites of infection, each virus type has a very restricted niche or site of infection, and the lesions caused by these viruses are usually benign. Phylogenetic studies suggest that viruses which occupy similar niches are also related genetically (*Figure 3.1*).

In normal, benign HPV-induced lesions, the cells contain HPV DNA in the form of circular episomes. The genome of the HPV-16 virus (*Figure 3.2*), is comprised of a long control region (LCR), necessary for normal virus replication and control of gene expression, and open reading frames divided into early (E) and late (L) genes. The E1 and E2 genes are involved in viral replication and transcriptional control [2], the E6 and E7 proteins inhibit the activity of negative regulators of the cell cycle and are discussed in Section 3.5, and the late open reading frames L1 and L2 encode structural proteins. Despite its position in the early region of the genome, the E4 gene accumulates within the cell at the same time as the late proteins. The function of the E4 protein is unknown although it has been shown to associate with cytokeratins and has been suggested to enhance virus release from the cell [3]. The E5 gene encodes the major transforming protein of bovine papillomavirus (BPV) type 1 which appears to function by interacting with cell surface growth factor receptors and transmitting a proliferative signal [4,5]. Although quite dissimilar from the BPV E5 at the amino acid level there is some evidence that the HPV E5

*Viruses and Human Cancer*, edited by J.R. Arrand and D.R. Harper

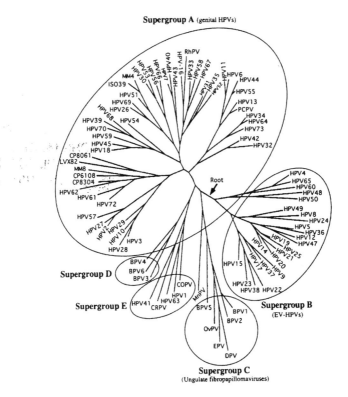

**Figure 3.1.** A phylogenetic tree of 92 papillomavirus types based on DNA sequence analysis of a 291 base pair segment of the L1 major capsid protein gene. For further details of this method of analysis and HPV phylogeny see [1]. Reproduced with permission of the American Society for Microbiology, from Chan *et al.*, 1995, Journal of Virology Vol. 69.

proteins may be functionally similar.

The papillomaviruses have been demonstrated to play a causal role in carcinogenesis in animals and overwhelming evidence suggests that HPV are involved in cancer in humans, most notably squamous cell carcinoma of the anogenital tract [6]. The mechanisms by which these viruses contribute to malignant progression are becoming understood, and a wealth of data on the activity of the viral oncoproteins has provided compelling evidence implicating these viruses in the pathogenesis of these cancers.

## 3.2 HPV and skin cancer

Infection by most types of cutaneous papillomaviruses generally results in nothing more than benign warts. However in some relatively rare instances there appears to be a relationship between certain papillomaviruses and skin cancer (see Section 1.3).

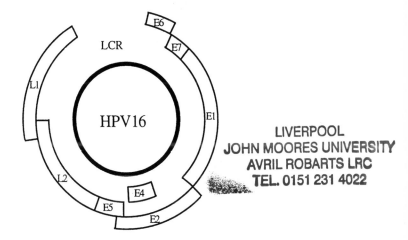

**Figure 3.2.** HPV–16 genome structure. The open reading frames are represented by open boxes.

The rare, life-long skin disease known as epidermodysplasia verruciformis (EV) is a multifactorial condition which is specifically associated with certain types of HPV, in particular HPV-5, -8, -9, -12, -14, -15, -17 and -19 – 25 [7]. A large proportion of these patients develop skin carcinomas which frequently harbour the genome of HPV-5 or 8.

An increasingly more common occurrence of skin carcinoma is found in renal transplant patients. As with EV, the associated HPV is predominantly type 5 or 8 and cancer development appears to be associated with long-term immunosuppression [8]. In contrast to the situation in cervical carcinoma (see below) the viral genome in HPV-associated skin carcinomas appears to be maintained in an episomal form. These virus types also appear to have different transformation strategies when compared with the mucoepitheliotropic genital papillomaviruses (below). In particular neither HPV-5 nor HPV-8 encodes an E5 polypeptide, the HPV-8 E6 gene appears not to form complexes with p53 and finally, HPV-8 E7 does not bind to the cellular retinoblastoma (RB) protein [9].

Research into the details of the potential roles of these viruses in the induction and maintenance of these skin carcinomas has lagged considerably behind corresponding efforts in connection with cervical carcinoma. The remainder of this chapter concentrates on this latter situation.

## 3.3 Epidemiological evidence for the involvement of HPV in cervical cancer

The identification of cancer of the cervix as a sexually transmitted disease was first made in 1834 and the hypothesis that HPV was involved in the generation of cervical cancer was suggested in the mid-1970s [10]. However, strong epidemiological data linking HPV with human cancer have been obtained only relatively recently. Studies have demonstrated that the majority of cervical cancers are HPV-positive and that only certain HPV types are correlated with invasive carcinoma, whereas other types are found predominantly in benign lesions. Many studies have attempted to distinguish the important differences between the cancer-associated or high-risk HPV types, most commonly HPV-16 and HPV-18, and the low-risk HPV types found almost exclusively in benign lesions, the most common being HPV-6 and HPV-11.

There are a number of difficulties in the design of epidemiological surveys, which have complicated the interpretation of these studies. One problem lies in the variability in the methods used for the detection of HPV infection. Most studies assay for the presence of DNA, by either DNA hybridization techniques or employing consensus primers allowing detection of the majority of HPV types by polymerase chain reaction (PCR) assays. The latter method is particularly sensitive and gives a much higher incidence of infection than when a hybridization approach is applied, but the sensitivity also can result in the identification of falsely positive samples. The exact incidence of HPV infection in the general population as detected by PCR was at first controversial, although recent studies show much more agreement.

The peak of HPV prevalence is at around 25 years of age, with the levels of infection decreasing with increased age after this point. This infection profile has been suggested to be the result of exposure to viral infection following the onset of sexual activity, and the decreased levels with age the result of an acquired immunity. An alternative explanation is that the increased levels of infection in young women are the result of an overall increase in the amount of HPV infections, potentially leading to a significant increase in cervical cancer in the future. As there is no serological assay to detect past exposure to HPV infection, it is difficult to correlate the differences in HPV infection to immune clearance or increased viral exposure. These alternative explanations illustrate the difficulty of analysing data in the form of a cross-sectional analysis of the population. A more informative approach is the use of prospective cohort studies, in which defined groups of women are studied over a period of time. This allows the analysis of the length of time following initial infection to progression to a higher grade lesion. Dysplastic lesions of the cervical epithelium are classified as cervical intraepithelial neoplasia (CIN) grade I, II and III, with CIN I representing mild dysplasia and CIN III representing severe dysplasia. Implicit in the classification is the notion of progression from low- to high-grade CIN and eventually fully malignant carcinoma, although many low-grade lesions naturally regress and generally have normal karyotypes whereas the higher grade CIN is aneuploid and has a higher chance of malignant progression.

The presence of HPV DNA can be detected by hybridization at a 5–10-fold higher frequency than cytological abnormalities. Patients who are HPV-positive by DNA detection, are often HPV-negative on a second examination several months later. However, it is unclear whether loss or appearance of detectable HPV DNA is the result of new infection/clearance or the result of persistent chronic infection. Although there is controversy as to what constitutes a clinical HPV infection, persistent levels of HPV DNA detectable by Southern blot is likely to be the most significant in terms of the risk of cancer development and infection with high-risk HPV types is clearly the major risk factor identified so far in the development of cervical cancer [11]. Other risk factors have been implicated in the development of cervical cancer, including smoking, use of oral contraceptives, young age of first sexual experience and a high number of sexual partners. However, the data are conflicting, and it is unclear whether these differences are the result of different populations used in different studies. Genital HPV-infection has also been associated with cancers other than cervical, including cancers of the penis, vulva and anus. Although there is strong evidence of a role of viral infection in these diseases, it is unclear why they are relatively less common than cancer of the cervix, despite similar levels of HPV infection. Data have also linked HPV DNA to a number of cancers of the oral cavity, digestive and respiratory tracts. Although there is no strong epidemiological evidence, at present, implicating HPV as a major risk factor in the development of these cancers, it seems likely that HPV infection plays a role in a subset of these tumours.

## 3.4 Transforming and immortalizing functions of HPVs

The use of *in vitro* assays to test genes for the ability to alter the properties of cells in culture has provided a powerful tool for the evaluation of the properties of oncogenes. The ability of genes to extend the life span of cells in culture indefinitely is termed immortalization. Although this measures an increased proliferation capacity of a cell, this is not the same as full transformation, which requires the acquisition of at least some of the properties characteristic of fully malignant cells. These include the ability to grow to a high saturation density, loss of contact inhibition, reduced growth factor requirements and growth in an anchorage-independent manner. The most stringent test for full transformation is the ability to generate tumours when introduced into nude mice.

Transforming and immortalizing activities of HPV DNA were initially demonstrated in rodent cells and subsequently it has been shown that HPV-16 and HPV-18 can immortalize primary human keratinocytes (which resemble the normal target cell of the virus) without obvious morphological transformation [12]. Further work comparing the ability of DNA from high-risk (HPV-16 and HPV-18) to that of low-risk viruses (HPV-6 and HPV-11) for the ability to immortalize human keratinocytes revealed that unlike the high risk viruses, low risk viruses do not alter the lifespan of transfected human cells, which senesce at the same rate as non-transfected cells [13]. Similarly, the low risk viruses perform poorly in the transformation of rodent cells in comparison with the high-risk virus types.

Analysis of the viral genome revealed that only the E6 and E7 open reading frames were necessary for the transformation of rodent cells and the immortalization of human genital keratinocytes [14,15]. Although E7 can function alone in human genital keratinocyte immortalization assays when placed under the control of a powerful promoter, E6 is required when E7 is under normal viral control, indicating a role for both of these proteins in immortalization. E6 alone is unable to immortalize primary human genital keratinocytes but can function alone in mammary-derived epithelial cells [16], illustrating the importance of cell-specific factors in the outcome of these assays. Although some difference between high- and low-risk viruses in the ability to function in immortalization and transformation assays may be due to differences in the level of expression of the E6 and E7 open reading frames, there is convincing evidence that the major difference is due to functional differences in the proteins themselves (see Section 3.5).

Although primary human keratinocytes immortalized by the HPV E6/E7 oncogenes show an extended lifespan, they do not display other characteristics of transformed cells, such as anchorage independence, and are incapable of inducing tumours in nude mice. These immortalized cell lines do, however, show abnormalities in differentiation. Alterations in differentiation are most clearly illustrated when cells are grown under organotypic culture conditions, (raft culture) where epithelial cells stratify and show morphology and differentiation similar to that seen *in vivo*. Using this system, HPV-16 and HPV-18-infected primary human keratinocytes exhibit a differentiation pattern which is almost indistinguishable from low-grade CIN [17], a premalignant lesion which normally contains HPV DNA. This work was extended to demonstrate that E6 and E7 were both necessary and sufficient for alteration of normal epithelial differentiation. The raft culture has also illustrated that low-grade CIN lesions and invasive squamous cell carcinoma can be mimicked successfully *in vitro*, by transferring clinical material to raft cultures. The observation that HPV-infected cultures of primary human keratinocytes can induce CIN-like lesions in raft culture, and the presence of HPV in these lesions *in vivo* strongly supports a causal role for HPV in the induction of these premalignant lesions.

It is clear that infection of cells with high-risk HPV types is not sufficient to induce tumorigenesis, as illustrated by the fact that carcinoma development is rare compared with the incidence of HPV infection. In addition, a lag period of many years is necessary for a CIN lesion to progress to a carcinoma, and the majority of these lesions do not progress. These *in vivo* observations are mirrored *in vitro*, where HPV-immortalized primary human epithelial cells are not tumorigenic. Clearly other genetic events are necessary for the progression to malignant disease. Although HPV immortalized keratinocytes are not transformed, continued passage can allow conversion to a tumorigenic phenotype at low frequency. This passaging *in vitro* is associated with an increase in chromosomal abnormalities and a progressive alteration in differentiation properties, this leads to a loss of stratification in raft cultures, reflecting the changes seen in progression to invasive squamous cell carcinoma [18].

## 3.5 Function of the viral oncoproteins

### *3.5.1 E7*

The HPV E7 proteins are small, nuclear proteins which bind zinc via two cysteine motifs at the carboxyl-terminus (*Figure 3.3*), and the HPV-18 E7 has been shown to be capable of dimerizing via this motif. The papillomavirus E7 proteins show no structural similarity to any known cellular proteins, but they do show limited sequence similarity to oncoproteins encoded by other DNA tumour viruses, such as SV40 and adenovirus (Ad). A region in the amino ter-minus of E7 shows similarity to Ad E1A conserved region 2 (CR2) and simian virus 40 (SV40) large T (LT) antigen [19]. The very extreme amino terminus of E7 also shows limited similarity with Ad E1A conserved region 1 (CR1). In addition to this structural similarity, these proteins all show functional similar-ities including the ability to transactivate the Ad E2 promoter, induce DNA synthesis in quiescent cells and to co-operate with ras in transformation assays.

The immortalizing and transforming activities displayed by E7, Ad E1A and SV40 LT are dependent, at least in part, on their interactions with the product of the retinoblastoma susceptibility gene (pRB) [20]. pRB has a role in controlling cell division, and targeting of this protein by viral oncogenes can allow cells to escape some of the normal checks on proliferation. This role of E7 in inhibiting the function of pRB is supported by a study examining the status of the *RB-1* gene in HPV-positive and HPV-negative cervical carcinoma cell lines. This study revealed *RB-1* mutation in HPV-negative, but not in HPV-positive cells [21], suggesting that the abrogation of pRB function is a common event in cervical cancer, and this can be achieved either by somatic mutation or by HPV E7 expression.

The pRB tumour suppressor protein can block cell cycle progression at the G1/S boundary [22]. This activity is regulated by phosphorylation throughout the cell cycle, hypophosphorylated pRB being present in G0 and G1 and

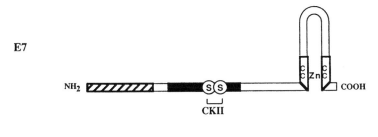

Region of similarity between E7 and E1A

Region of similarity between E7 and both E1A and LT. The region is responsible for the binding of pRB and contains a casein kinase II phosphorylation site.

**Figure 3.3.** The structure of the HPV–16 E7 protein.

phosphorylation at multiple sites by cyclin-dependent kinases occurring at the G1/S phase boundary. Hyperphosphorylated pRB is present in S, G2 and M phase, and dephosphorylation of pRB occurs late in M phase by the action of a phosphatase. The hypophosphorylated form of pRB, which is thought to act as a negative regulator of the cell cycle, binds to a number of transcription factors, most notably the E2F family. The E2F family of transcription factors is a critical mediator of cell cycle progression, controlling the expression of a number of genes involved in replication and cell cycle control, such as dihydrofolate reductase and DNA polymerase $\alpha$ and cyclin E [23]. Expression of the E2F-1 transcription factor in quiescent fibroblasts is sufficient to induce DNA synthesis, illustrating the central role of these transcription factors in the control of cell proliferation. Following cyclin dependent kinase phosphorylation of pRB, these transcription factors are released from pRB, allowing them to mediate transcriptional activation and progression through the G1/S boundary (*Figure 3.4*). pRB functions as a negative regulator of E2F in G1, acting by direct binding of the E2F transactivation domain. The viral oncoproteins E7, SV40 LT and Ad E1A circumvent this negative regulation via binding to hypophosphorylated pRB, displacing E2F and allowing cells to progress into S phase in the absence of normal mitogenic signals [24]. Induction of E7 expression in serum-starved fibroblasts can induce DNA synthesis and the ability of E7 to bind to pRB is essential for this activity, implying that it is mediated by E2F. The pRB-related p107 and p130 proteins also bind E2F transcription factors and show a similar ability to regulate transcriptional activity negatively. Although they are related, there is evidence that these proteins may regulate the expression of different genes, possibly as a result of differences in affinity for different E2F family members. In addition they may play a role at different stages of the cell cycle with p130 complexes predominating in quiescent cells. The function of E7 appears to involve the interference of the normal growth regulatory function of all the pRB protein family members.

Mutational analysis of the HPV-16 E7 has been extremely useful in unravelling the functions of this protein. This work has illustrated that CR2 is necessary for the ability to bind the pRB family members and a point mutation which abolishes this interaction renders this mutant transformation-defective. Single amino acid substitutions in this region have demonstrated that the binding of pRB and p107/p130 are separable and a point mutant which retains the ability to bind to p107/p130 but not pRB is transformation-defective, suggesting that targeting pRB may play a more important role in transformation, which is also indicated by the lack of mutations in either p107 or p130 genes in tumour cells. Sequences in the carboxyl-terminus of E7 have also been implicated in the functional consequences of the pRB–E7 interaction. Truncations of E7 abolish the ability of this protein to inhibit non-specific interaction of pRB with DNA and the ability of E7 to disrupt the E2F–pRB interaction requires carboxyl-terminal amino acids.

Targeting pRB is a common theme in DNA tumour virus strategy, and the

## E7 activates cell cycle progression by targeting pRB

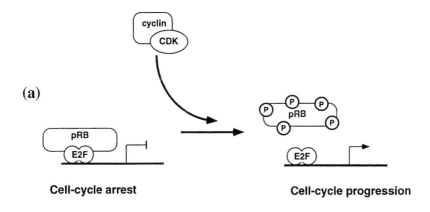

**(a)**

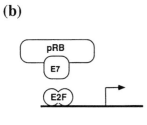

**Cell-cycle arrest**

**Cell-cycle progression**

**(b)**

**Cell-cycle progression**

**Figure 3.4.** (a) Normal control of E2F-mediated transcription by pRB. In G1, pRB binds to E2F rendering it transcriptionally inactive. At the G1/S boundary, pRB becomes phosphorylated and releases E2F which becomes transcriptionally active. (b) An E7-expressing cell always maintains free E2F as E7 binds pRB releasing E2F.

consequent deregulation of E2F transcription preventing a G1/S block could be proposed to extend the proliferative capacity of HPV-infected cells. Although this is an appealing model for the role of E7 in immortalization and transformation, there are a number of caveats. An E7 mutant which is significantly impaired in the ability to complex with pRB, when placed in the context of the whole virus genome, is still capable of immortalizing human epithelial cells despite the absolute requirement of E7 for this property [25]. Interestingly, the pRB binding activity is still important when only E6 and E7 are used and it seems likely that another function of HPV-16, as yet unidentified, can substitute for the pRB-binding activity of E7 in the immortalization of human epithelial cells. Similarly, the cottontail rabbit papillomavirus containing a mutation in the E7 gene which abolishes pRB interaction is still capable of inducing papillomas [26]. It should be remembered that immortalization and papilloma formation represent processes different from that of tumorigenesis. The binding of pRB is likely to play a role *in vivo* in the generation of cancer, given that this property is necessary for the E7-mediated transformation of rodent cells. It will be of great interest to determine whether the warts induced by the pRB non-binding virus are capable of progressing to full malignancy with the same efficiency as those induced by the wild-type virus.

Recent work has suggested that rather than simply inhibiting pRB family member function by competitive binding, E7 promotes their degradation [27, 28]. E7-expressing cells have lower levels of pRB protein and although the mechanism mediating this degradation is unknown, it is thought to involve the proteosome pathway. An E7 mutant incapable of binding to pRB was significantly impaired in the ability to induce its degradation, suggesting that the degradation could be mediated by a direct association. Interestingly, an amino-terminal mutation of E7 renders it incompetent in transformation and immortalization and although it is still being capable of binding to pRB it is significantly impaired in its ability to induce pRB degradation. This result suggests that the degradation, rather than simply competitive binding is important in the ability of E7 to transform cells.

E7 is involved in inducing cells to enter S phase via its interaction with pRB and related proteins. There is some evidence also that E7 can function later in the cell cycle, inducing cells to pass through G2 and enter mitosis. Immunoprecipitation studies have demonstrated that E7 has associated kinase activity, which has been identified as being mediated by a cyclin-dependent kinase with associated cyclin A or cyclin E. This kinase activity is at its highest in G2 suggesting that it may play a role at this stage of the cell cycle and sequences necessary for association with p107 and p130 are required for association with this kinase activity.

Further evidence of a potential role for E7 beyond simply binding to pRB is provided by studies of the ability of E7 to circumvent p53-mediated growth arrest pathways. Activation of p53 leads to both a G1 and a G2 arrest in RKO cells and expression of E7 allows these cells to traverse both of these cell cycle check points [29]. The E7-expressing cells still produce the cyclin-dependent kinase inhibitor p21$^{Waf1/Cip1}$ in response to p53, and it is functionally active. However, despite inhibition of overall cyclin-dependent kinase activity, these cells retain hyperphosphorylated pRB. Recent studies have suggested that the cyclin-dependent kinase which associates with E7 is resistant to inhibition by p21$^{Waf1/Cip1}$ [29], and since this kinase can phosphorylate pRB *in vitro*, it is possible that phosphorylation of pRB *in vivo* is also carried out by this kinase. Other studies have also suggested that E7 may be capable of directly binding to and inhibiting the function of p21$^{Waf1/Cip1}$.

In addition to the pRB binding domain of E7, other regions have been shown to contribute to the transformation of rodent cells, including the two phosphorylated serine residues in the casein kinase II site adjacent to the pRB binding site. Both E1A and E7 show evidence of mediating E2F-independent transcriptional activity. Some of the transcriptional functions of E1A are related to the interaction with p300, a cellular transcriptional co-activator, although there is no evidence that E7 can interact with this protein. Both E1A and E7 have been shown to be capable of interacting with the TATA-binding protein (TBP), the DNA binding component of the basal transcription complex TFIID, and $TAF_{II}110$, a TBP-associated cofactor, suggesting a possible mechanism of mediating transactivation of gene expression via interaction with these important components of the basal transcriptional machinery.

An indication of the significance of the various functions of E7 to tumorigenesis can be deduced from a comparative analysis of proteins encoded by the high- and low-risk viral types. The E7 proteins from high- and low-risk viruses show a number of biochemical and functional differences which could relate to the difference in oncogenic potential of the viral types from which they were derived. The E7 proteins from HPV-6 and HPV-11 bind pRB with a low affinity, transform rodent cells very poorly, are inefficient at immortalizing human epithelial cells and provide a poorer substrate for casein kinase II phosphorylation. Comparison of the sequence of the high-risk and low-risk E7 proteins revealed a single amino acid consistently different in the pRB-binding domain. Mutation of this residue revealed that this amino acid was the major determinant in the differences between high- and low-risk pRB-binding affinity and the transformation activity in rodent cells. Although the high-risk E7 proteins are a better substrate for CKII phosphorylation than the low risk, domain swap experiments failed to reveal any functional differences between these domains. One similarity between the high- and low-risk E7 proteins is the ability to transactivate the E2 promoter, suggesting that pRB interaction is not required for this function, perhaps being mediated by p107/p130 interaction.

### 3.5.2 E6

The HPV E6 protein is approximately 150 amino acids in length and contains four cysteine motifs (*Figure 3.5*), which are thought to be involved in zinc binding. There are no regions of detectable sequence similarity with either cellular protein or proteins from other DNA tumour viruses. However, the high-risk HPV E6 proteins show functional similarities with Ad E1B 55K and SV40 LT in that all three viral proteins bind to the cellular p53 protein and inhibit its

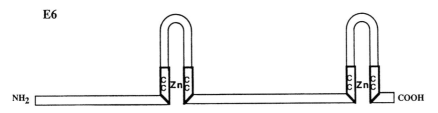

**Figure 3.5.** The structure of the HPV-16 E6 protein.

activity [30]. Unlike the other viral proteins, which induce a stabilization of p53, the high risk HPV E6 proteins target p53 for degradation via a ubiquitin-dependent pathway [31].

The p53 gene is a negative regulator of cell growth. Unlike the pRB family, this protein is not a constitutive component of cell cycle control, but is induced in response to DNA damage, inducing a G1 arrest and/or apoptosis [32]. The p53 protein is a transcription factor and is thought to mediate G1 arrest via the induction of the p21$^{Waf1/Cip1}$ gene which encodes an inhibitor of cyclin-dependent kinases (whose activities are necessary for cell cycle progression) [33]. The p53 gene is the most commonly mutated gene in human cancer [34], and loss of its activity may be generated by deletion or mutation resulting in the expression of an altered protein. Like SV40 LT and Ad E1B, the introduction of E6 into cells interferes with the DNA binding and transcription activity of p53.

Although degradation of p53 by E6 *in vitro* is very efficient, *in vivo* the levels of p53 in HPV E6 immortalized cells or in HPV-positive carcinomas are on average only two to three-fold lower than in normal primary cells and the half-life of p53 is decreased from 3 h to 20 min on the introduction of E6 into primary human keratinocytes. Interestingly, however, cells expressing E6 fail to mount a p53 induction in response to DNA damage [35] (*Figure 3.6*), suggesting that E6 may maintain p53 below a certain threshold level, or specifically degrade certain forms of p53.

The ubiquitin pathway of protein degradation has been well characterized [36]. Ubiquitin is a small 76 amino acid peptide which has been identified in

**(a)**    p53 induces cell cycle arrest and apoptosis

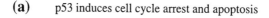

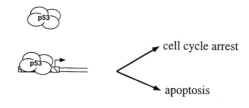

**(b)**    E6 expressing cell

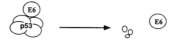

cell cycle progression

**Figure 3.6. (a)** p53 induces cell cycle arrest and apoptosis. **(b)** In an E6 expressing cell, p53 fails to induce either cell cycle arrest or apoptosis as a result of the E6-mediated degradation of p53.

all eukaryotic organisms. A cascade of reactions results in the transfer of ubiquitin to the target protein. These ubiquitin molecules themselves can be ubiquitinated leading to the formation of a multi-ubiquitinated protein, which is recognized by a proteosome complex and degraded. Studies of p53–E6 interactions have led to the identification of a large protein which binds E6 and p53 in a complex, termed the E6-associated protein or E6-AP. This protein is required for the E6-mediated degradation and the ubiquitination of p53 and the data suggest that the E6–E6-AP complex functions as an ubiquitin-ligase which may be involved in the regulation of a number of different proteins in both normal and E6-transformed cells [37]. It will be of great interest to determine if the interaction between E6 and E6-AP mediates the degradation of other proteins which regulate normal cell growth.

Loss of wild-type p53 function clearly plays a role in the development of most human tumours and p53 has been suggested to act as the 'guardian of the genome' [38], inducing growth arrest or apoptosis in response to DNA damage and thus protecting the cell from replication of unrepaired DNA. Strong evidence supporting the importance of the targeting of the p53 protein by E6 in tumorigenesis is provided by analysis of the distribution of mutations of this gene in tumours. Mutations in the p53 gene are very common in almost all solid tumours, with the exception of anogenital cancer [21,39]. The striking absence of p53 mutations in HPV-positive cervical tumours supports the role for E6 in inactivating p53 function at the level of the protein, alleviating the necessity for the selection of somatic mutation within the p53 gene during tumour development.

Initial comparisons of E6 proteins from different viral types indicated that E6 from low-risk viruses was incapable of interacting with p53 or promoting its degradation. These observations provided an attractive model for the difference in the ability of low- and high-risk HPV types to contribute to carcinogenesis where interference of p53 function by E6 may lead to the accumulation of genetic alterations, potentially contributing to oncogenic progression. An inability of low-risk E6 proteins to inhibit p53 activity would allow cells infected with these viruses to undergo a normal physiological response to DNA damage, with an accompanying genome stability lacking in those cells infected with high-risk virus. The situation is probably complex however, and there is evidence that the low-risk E6 proteins do retain some ability to bind p53 and interfere with DNA binding, albeit less efficiently than the high-risk E6 proteins. These results suggest that the difference between high-risk and low-risk E6 may be quantitative rather than qualitative with respect to abrogation of p53 function and several *in vivo* studies have described low but detectable activities for low-risk E6 proteins in abrogating p53 transcription functions and immortalization of human keratinocytes.

Clearly the targeting of p53 for degradation is an important function for both the normal viral life cycle and the generation of a tumour. However, in addition to this function of E6, other activities may contribute to the immortalization and/or transforming properties of this oncoprotein. Recent work has implicated the E6 oncoprotein from the high-risk viruses in activating telomerase, which could be a potentially important mechanism of HPV-mediated immortalization [40]. Mammalian telomeres are long structures consisting of multiple repeats of TTAGG, which shorten as a function of division *in vivo* as a consequence of an intrinsic inability to replicate the 3' end of DNA. Normal primary cells, when grown in culture, divide until the telomeres reach a critical length signalling senescence, this is termed the M1 block. E6- and E7-expressing cells can escape this senescence and continue to proliferate, with consequent further shortening of the telomeres. These cells eventually reach crisis (or M2) presumably as a result of chromosome instability and the majority of the population dies. The cells which emerge from crisis have stabilized telomeres, and very commonly activated telomerase. Telomerase is an enzyme which replaces the telomeric repeats and is not normally expressed in somatic cells. Activation of telomerase is a common event in the generation of cell lines and tumours, presumably allowing cells to escape from the senescence signalled by telomeric shortening.

Expression of E6 in keratinocytes was sufficient to induce telomerase activity (although not in all cells in the culture), and this induction of telomerase activity could be detected on early passage after viral infection, indicating that it is a direct consequence of E6 expression rather than a rare genetic event. Although expression of E7 was not required for the induction of telomerase, it was necessary for immortalization indicating that the ability of E6 to induce telomerase activity is not sufficient for immortalization. Mutant E6 incapable of binding to p53 retains full wild-type activity for the activation of telomerase, indicating that this activity is p53 independent. Interestingly this mutant was still capable of binding to E6-AP, suggesting the intriguing possibility that E6 may mediate this function by targeting degradation of an unknown protein, perhaps one that is responsible for negatively regulating telomerase activity. Although E6 can activate telomerase, this does not result in the stabilization of telomere lengths in these cultures, and E7-expressing cells alone can partially restore telomere length at late passage, without detectable telomerase activity [41]. This suggests that there must be E6- and perhaps telomerase-independent mechanisms to stabilize telomere length. The importance of this function of E6 in HPV-induced immortalization and transformation is unclear at present although, interestingly, low-risk E6 shows a greatly impaired ability to induce telomerase activity as compared with high-risk E6.

Other, as yet unknown, functions may also contribute to the transforming or immortalizing activities of E6. The existence of other activities is suggested by transformation assays in rodent cells, in which mutant p53 is unable to substitute functionally for E6 and there is some evidence that E6 can block certain forms of apoptosis in a p53-independent manner [42]. It is interesting to note that an E6 binding protein has been identified which has sequence homology to calcium binding proteins [43]. Although the role of this interaction in HPV-mediated functions awaits further experimentation, the importance of calcium in keratinocyte differentiation suggests intriguing possibilities. Another apparently p53-independent property of the E6 protein is its ability to transactivate the expression of a number of heterologous promoters, including 'minimal' TATA containing promoters [44]. How this activity is mediated is unknown, but it is unlikely to be involved in transformation as both high- and low-risk E6 proteins share this property.

### 3.5.3 Function of E6 and E7 in non–transformed cells

The work described here has outlined how the interaction between the HPV proteins and cellular regulators of cell growth may contribute to the generation of cancer. Clearly this is not the normal function of these proteins in the viral

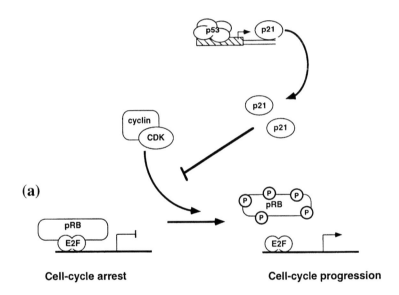

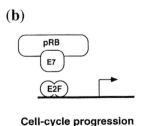

**Figure 3.7. (a)** Normal cell cycle arrest mediated in response to DNA damage. p53 is stabilized on DNA damage and transcriptionally activates the p21$^{Waf1/Cip1}$ gene; p21$^{Waf1/Cip1}$ inhibits the cyclin-dependent kinase mediated phosphorylation of pRB, blocking the cells in G1. **(b)** In an E7-expressing cell, p21$^{Waf1/Cip1}$-induced growth arrest is subverted by release of free E2F as a result of E7/pRB interaction.

life cycle. Detailed analysis of normal HPV replication has been difficult due to the inability to culture virus to high titres successfully *in vitro*. However, many aspects have been studied using organotypic raft culture and analysis of naturally occurring lesions *in situ*.

HPV infect the basal epithelium, which is the dividing layer of this tissue. As cells move upwards, they normally cease dividing and differentiate. Analysis of cervical lesions has revealed that viral replication occurs in layers of cells which would not normally be dividing. As the HPV does not encode its own replication machinery, it is necessary for the virus to maintain the cell in a state which is capable of replicating the viral genome. The viral strategy appears to be to prevent checks to cell cycle progression to promote increased proliferation rather than differentiation. It is tempting to speculate that the function of E7 is to release E2F from pRB, irrespective of the normal cell cycle controls, to induce abnormal cellular DNA synthesis. However, it must be remembered that cottontail rabbit papillomavirus (CRPV) E7 is still able to induce warts when mutated such that it cannot interact with pRB, indicating that this activity is not necessary for the induction of benign lesions.

The detection of viral replication within the cell as DNA damage, with consequent induction of p53 activity, may explain the normal role of E6 in targeting p53. Although E6 might be necessary to abrogate the p53-mediated growth arrest, recent understanding of the mechanism of p53 function has suggested that E7, like E6, should be capable of bypassing this G1 arrest (*Figure 3.7*) [45]. Briefly, p53 is stabilized following DNA damage and this directly activates expression of the wild-type p53 activated fragment 1/cyclin dependent kinase interacting protein 1 ($p21^{Waf1/Cip1}$) gene. The $p21^{Waf1/Cip1}$ protein inhibits the activity of the cyclin dependent kinases, which prevents phosphorylation of pRB and hence inhibits the release of E2F, blocking cells in G1 (but see Section 6.5.9 for an alternative interpretation of $p21^{Waf1/Cip1}$ function). This effect, however, would be predicted to be bypassed by the action of E7 which binds to hypophosphorylated pRB releasing E2F. Indeed, cells expressing E7 have been demonstrated to be resistant to p53-induced G1 growth arrest following DNA damage [46]. The importance of E6 to tumour development (and most probably to the normal viral life cycle), may be in abrogating the apoptotic rather than the growth arrest function of p53. Although perturbation and activation of E2F function by E7 will promote cell-cycle progression, deregulated E2F expression in the presence of p53 also elicits a strong apoptotic effect [47]. In the absence of a mechanism to inactivate p53, expression of E7 may simply result in cell death, a hypothesis which has been elegantly supported by studies utilizing transgenic mice [48]. Targeted expression of HPV-16 E7 gives rise to degenerate lesions with evidence of apoptosis, a phenotype which is dependent on the pRB binding activity of E7. This effect was shown to be mediated by p53, as similar transgenic mice in a p53 null background or double transgenics containing the E6 and E7 genes showed a reduced level of apoptosis. These results demonstrate that E7 expression can induce apoptosis via a p53-dependent pathway, which can be abrogated by E6, and support the notion that a normal function of the E6 protein is to block the apoptotic signal generated by E7. The relative differences in the strengths of the high- and low-risk E6 ability to abrogate p53 function may be a response to the much lower affinity of low-risk E7 for pRB. Consequently, a weaker apoptotic signal may be generated by low-risk E7 in comparison to that generated by the high-risk E7 proteins, and it would be of interest to determine whether the low-risk E7 proteins are capable of inducing apoptosis in the transgenic models.

### 3.5.4 E5

The principal transforming oncoprotein of BPV is the E5 oncoprotein. In contrast, HPV E5 has only weakly transforming properties. Although high-risk HPV E5 is unable to immortalize keratinocytes, it is able to enhance immortalization [49], induce anchorage-independent growth of mouse fibroblasts and stimulate the growth of rat kidney cells in co-operation with E7 [50]. This gene is not consistently maintained in fully malignant cervical cancer and is therefore unlikely to play a role in the maintenance of the transformed phenotype. E5 is a small membrane-bound protein that associates with cell surface receptors such as the platelet-derived growth factor receptor and the epidermal growth factor (EGF) receptor, and inhibits the down-regulation of the receptor in the presence of ligand, resulting in an increased level of receptor on the cell surface, and is able to enhance the transforming activity of the EGF receptor [51]. E5 has been shown to bind to a component of the vacuolar $H^+$-ATPases [52] and decreases gap junctional communication, which may function to make cells unresponsive to growth control signals from adjoining cells [53]. Although expression of the E5 gene is often lost on integration of the papillomavirus genome into cellular DNA, given its *in vitro* transforming functions and sequence similarity to BPV-1 E5, it is possible that E5 plays a role in the early stages of malignant progression. It should be noted that although the BPV-4 virus is a causative agent in the induction of alimentary canal cancer in cattle, viral DNA is not usually retained in the fully invasive carcinoma, or in cells which have been transformed with BPV-4 oncoproteins, despite the viral oncogenes being essential for this transformation [54]. The BPV-4 viral DNA must presumably act by a 'hit and run' mechanism, and not be required for the maintenance of the transformed cell. It is possible that HPV E5 could function in a similar fashion.

## 3.6 Progression to the full malignant phenotype

As with other tumour viruses (see Sections 1.3, 2.7 and 4.9), simple infection by high-risk HPV is not sufficient for full malignant transformation, and increasing effort is being directed into understanding the events which contribute to malignant progression. Detectable HPV infection has been shown to follow an age-dependent distribution, peaking in women in their early 20s, presumably as they become sexually active. A steady decline in HPV infection with increasing age suggests immune clearance and it is possible that malignant progression is limited to those individuals with persistent infections.

Following infection with high risk HPV, factors which may influence progression to invasive carcinoma are likely to function by promoting one of the following:

(i)    evasion of host immunity; given the viral nature of the disease, persistence of infection is likely to be of great importance allowing time for other genetic events to take place;

(ii)    alteration of expression of the viral genes. Changes which result in the maximum levels of unregulated expression of the viral oncogenes are likely to induce tumorigenic changes, given the genetic instability they induce;

(iii)    accumulation of further genetic changes in the host's genome.

Factors which have been suggested to increase the risk of malignant progress are all likely to act via promoting one or more of the above categories of events, and for malignant carcinoma to occur it is likely that persistence of infection, deregulation of the viral oncogene expression and further genetic events, in addition to HPV infection are all required.

Animal studies have provided direct evidence for the role of co-factors in the generation of papillomavirus-positive cancer [55], with the first demonstration of the effect of co-carcinogens in the induction of tumours in cottontail rabbit with CRPV and chemical carcinogens in 1934. Other models include the BPV-4 which co-operates with carcinogens in bracken fern in the generation of alimentary tract cancer. Similar experiments with HPV-immortalized primary human keratinocytes demonstrated that treatment with nitrosomethylurea and 12-O-tetradecanoylphorbol-13-acetate (TPA) resulted in full tumorigenic conversion.

### 3.6.1 The role of immunity in HPV-induced  carcinogenesis

The development of cancer requires a number of genetic hits (see Section 1.3), explaining the increased incidence of cancer with age. Deregulation of the E2F and p53 pathways probably occur in all tumour types, and this deregulation leads to genetic instability and as a consequence increased likelihood of accumulating further genetic change required for the development of a fully invasive carcinoma. Infection with papillomavirus probably results in the functional equivalent of a number of genetic hits; however, persistent expression of the viral oncoproteins is necessary for the development of the tumour. As cervical cancer has a viral aetiology, the ability of the immune system to clear infection will greatly influence the probability of neoplastic progression, and persistent infection with HPV is associated with the greatest risk of developing high-grade CIN. A number of lines of evidence have suggested the importance of the immune system for the development of cervical cancer. Increased incidence of high-grade CIN following human immune deficiency virus (HIV) infection and an association of specific haplotypes of human leucocyte antigen type II with cervical cancer suggest the importance of cell-mediated immunity in the protection from HPV-induced cervical cancer. Other factors which have been epidemiologically linked to cervical cancer could have an effect on the ability of the host to control/eliminate papillomavirus. Multiple pregnancy, which results in a period of immunosuppression, showed an association with increased risk of cervical cancer, and is also associated with greater papillomavirus infection. Smoking is also considered a risk factor, and in addition to any mutagenic effects, there is evidence that it may produce an impaired immune response to genital papillomavirus infection. The loss of most viral DNA in carcinomas with the exception of the viral oncoproteins may reduce the immune response, as the structural proteins are immunogenic, and their expression is normally lost on progression to carcinoma (see below).

Experimental models have also demonstrated the role of the immune system in HPV- mediated cancer. The bracken which can act as a co-carcinogen in the development of BPV-4-associated tumours contains chemicals which are both immunosuppressive and mutagenic. The immunosuppressive effects lead to activation of latent virus which results in uncontrolled spread of the virus and the development of florid papillomatosis, and the normal process of papilloma rejection is impaired. This process greatly expands the pool of target cells on which the mutagenic factors in bracken can act.

### 3.6.2 The role of viral integration and deregulation of gene expression in tumorigenesis

Although HPV DNA, like Epstein–Barr virus (see Section 4.2), is maintained episomally in benign lesions, in anogenital cancers the viral DNA is most often integrated into the host genome [56], suggesting that, as with hepatitis B virus (see Section 2.4), integration plays a role in malignant progression. Although some studies have mapped sites of integration close to proto-oncogenes, there seems to be no preferred or specific site of integration (although the virus may preferentially integrate at chromosomal fragile sites), suggesting that the consequence of integration is not the alteration of the regulation or properties of a cellular gene. The integration event however, does show specificity with respect to the viral genome (*Figure 3.8*), consistently resulting in the disruption of E2 and E1 expression with frequent loss or mutation of open reading frames other than E6 and E7. As E2 can function as a repressor of E6 and E7 transcription, its loss contributes to the deregulated expression of these open reading frames [57]. The integration event can also result in the stabilization of E6/E7 mRNA, by inactivating a 3' destabilization sequence in the viral RNA. In addition to the escape from E2-mediated repression, some integration events may deregulate E6/E7 expression by placing these viral genes under the control of promoter sequences at the site of integration.

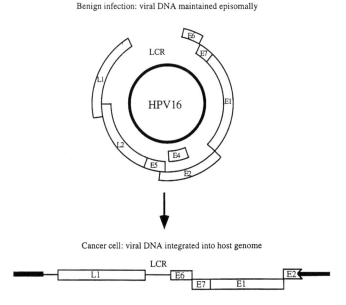

Figure 3.8. The effect of integration on the viral genome. Typically, the E2 open reading frame is disrupted, allowing escape from E2-mediated repression of the E6 and E7 open reading frames.

Loss of normal regulation of E6 and E7 expression can also occur by mechanisms other than viral integration. The viral LCR is regulated by a number of negatively acting cellular factors and the cellular YY1 protein has been shown to repress the activity of HPV transcription.

Mutations within the viral LCR, resulting in loss of YY1-mediated regulation of E6 and E7 expression, have been detected in several cancers showing evidence of only episomal viral DNA [58]. These results highlight the importance of deregulated E6 and E7 expression to both the development and the maintenance of the tumour. Indeed, there is evidence that the growth of HPV-associated cancer cells is dependent on continued E6 and E7 expression.

### 3.6.3 Role of steroid hormones in the progression of cervical cancer

Steroid hormones have been implicated in the development of cervical carcinoma, both by epidemiological and experimental approaches. Pregnancy appears to generate conditions which seem to allow persistent HPV infection which could be related to hormonal changes. Long-term use of oral contraceptives also has been implicated as a risk factor for the development of cervical cancer. Both pregnancy and oral contraceptives result in the alteration of the normal levels of progesterone and oestrogen in the body. Intriguingly, the site of most cervical carcinomas is the metaplastic epithelium, an area also responsive to steroid hormones.

The steroid hormones bind to their cognate receptors which then function directly as transcription factors. An attractive hypothesis for the action of the steroid hormones is that they affect the levels of the viral gene products directly. The LCR of HPV-16 has been shown to contain a progesterone–glucocorticoid-like responsive element, which mediates elevated transcription in response to steroid hormones. Elevated levels of steroids may therefore lead to increased persistence of infection and elevated risk of malignant progression.

Although it is possible that the elevation of HPV transcription contributes to the increased risk of cervical cancer associated with increased steroid hormone levels, not all cervical cancer cell lines show increased transcription in response to hormone. An alternative mechanism of action is increased cellular proliferation in response to high levels of oestrogen, since the cervical epithelium contains functional oestrogen receptors, potentially providing an expanded pool of cells available for malignant transformation.

A transgenic mouse model has provided evidence of a role for oestrogen as a co-operating factor with HPV in the generation of cervical cancer. Targeting expression of the HPV-16 early transcription region to the epidermis, using a K14 promoter, was used as a model of papillomavirus infection. Although the mice failed to develop tumours, chronic treatment of the mice with oestrogen led to 100% of the mice showing neoplastic progression in the squamous epithelium of the vagina and cervix, with 60% of the mice going on to develop fully invasive carcinoma [59]. As the viral LCR is not present and the K14 promoter is unresponsive to oestrogen, the development of carcinoma cannot simply be due to a direct up-regulation of viral transcription. Although there is a modest increase in the level of viral expression by some unknown indirect mechanism, it is unclear whether this up-regulation of oncoprotein expression is the mechanism of co-operation between oestrogen exposure and HPV early gene expression in this system.

### 3.6.4 The role of chromosome 11 in malignant progression

Cytogenetic studies have suggested that the loss of chromosome 11 may play a role in the development of cervical cancer. More direct evidence for the presence of a tumour suppressor gene(s) on chromosome 11 comes from studies showing that the loss of tumorigenicity of HPV-positive cervical carcinoma cell lines correlates with the introduction of a normal chromosome 11. The tumour suppressor gene on chromosome 11 has been suggested to function by repressing transcription of the HPV genome, as E6 and E7 expression is lost on the generation of tumour cell hybrids containing a normal chromosome 11 [60], and human embryo fibroblasts containing a deletion on chromosome 11 fail to show the repression of viral transcription which is seen in normal fibroblasts [61]. These results suggest normal cellular mechanisms exist to control viral gene expression, and that these may be deregulated during malignant progression. The identity of the putative tumour suppressor gene on chromosome 11 remains to be identified.

### 3.6.5 Other genetic events in the progression of cervical cancer

In addition to the deregulation of E6 and E7 expression, other genetic events are required before fully invasive carcinoma can manifest itself. As discussed earlier, although E6 and E7 can extend the life span of infected cells, immortalization is a rare event and still further genetic change is required before the cells become transformed.

The importance of genetic changes is reflected in the karyotype of different grades of CIN. Low grade CIN is generally diploid, whereas high grade CIN lesions characteristically are aneuploid and show karyotypic abnormalities. The genetic changes involved in progression to invasive carcinoma are likely to consist of both loss of tumour suppressor genes and activation of oncogenes. The evidence seems to suggest that, rather than acting as a true tumour suppressor, chromosome 11 mediates negative regulation of viral expression. However, other cytogenetic abnormalities have also been detected in cervical carcinoma specimens and in immortalized cells *in vitro*, which may represent classical tumour suppressor genes. These studies have suggested that loss of chromosomes 1, 3 and 5 may be involved in carcinogenesis of the cervix; one study revealed that 21 out of 47 cervical cancer samples showed loss of heterozygosity at one or more loci on chromosome 3p, the common region mapping to 3p13-p21.1, and loss of this region has also been reported in HPV-immortalized keratinocytes. This region has been demonstrated to be deleted in carcinomas of the lung, breast and kidney, suggesting that this region may encompass a novel tumour suppressor gene. Many other regions have also been implicated in various studies, both in carcinoma samples, cervical carcinoma cell lines or immortalized cells, suggesting that there may be many different aberrations potentially responsible for oncogenic progression. p53 mutations have also been identified in metastases derived from HPV-positive carcinomas [62], suggesting that expression of a mutant p53 protein may have different consequences than its loss following E6 degradation, and may contribute to malignant progression. There is considerable evidence that mutant p53 proteins acquire dominant transforming functions, even in p53 null cells [63].

In addition to the loss of tumour suppressor genes, the activation of oncogenes is likely to play a role. Mutations in *ets-2, erg, ras* and other oncogenes have been identified in both cancer samples and cell lines, however what role they play in the disease has yet to be determined. Oncogenes such as *ras* and *fos* have been demonstrated to be capable of co-operating with the HPV genome in the transformation of both human and rodent cells. Amplification of c-*myc*, or activation as a result of integration of the HPV genome are changes that have been suggested as playing a role in progression. It seems likely that a number of oncogenes could be involved in the progression to carcinoma, given that they have the ability to co-operate with E7 in converting immortalized lines to fully transformed lines.

In addition to the HPVs, several other genital tract infections have also been suggested as participating in malignant progression. Epidemiological evidence has implicated herpes simplex virus (HSV) infection in the generation of cervical cancer and *in vitro* experiments have shown that the HSV-2 genome has transforming functions. HPV-immortalized keratinocytes transfected with a fraction of the HSV-2 genome were capable of forming tumours in nude mice, although the HSV-2 sequences were lost, suggesting that HSV-2 acts via a 'hit and run' mechanism [64]. There is no strong evidence for the involvement of other sexually transmitted diseases, although preliminary evidence suggests that HIV infection results in a significantly higher incidence of CIN, with clear consequences for eventual risks of cancer development.

There are isolated reports of potential synergy between HPV and human T-cell leukemia virus type I (see Section 6.3.1.1).

## 3.7 Viral genes as targets for therapy

As cervical cancer has a viral component, this provides unique opportunities to develop therapeutic strategies which target the viral gene products. The most obvious strategy is the development of prophylactic or therapeutic vaccines. These are considered in Chapter 7.

In addition to vaccines, targeting the viral oncoproteins to inhibit their function directly is an alternative approach. A number of studies have demonstrated that continued expression of E6/E7 is necessary for tumour cell growth and antisense approaches have been shown to reduce expression of the viral oncoproteins in cervical cancer lines and abolish their tumorigenicity in nude mice [65]. Rather than targeting both E6 and E7, attempting to functionally inactivate E6 alone could be a better approach. The evasion of apoptosis is a necessary requirement of a tumour cell, and the functional inactivation of the apoptotic tumour suppressor gene p53 is one mechanism by which this can be achieved. E7 expression alone can generate a proliferative response via deregulating endogenous E2F activity. However, in the absence of E6 this results in apoptosis mediated at least in part by p53. Targeting of E6 in a cell expressing E7 would be predicted to provoke an apoptotic response as a result of elevating p53 levels. Experiments along these lines have been undertaken, and have shown, in principle, that this approach may be successful. Antisense experiments have targeted the endogenous E6-AP which is required for E6-mediated degradation of p53. This successfully lowered the levels of E6-AP and increased p53 levels only in E6-positive cells, suggesting that this could specifically affect tumour cells [66]. Interfering with E6 function is an attractive approach to the treatment of cervical cancer and could potentially be undertaken utilizing either a gene therapy protocol or by the development of small, cell permeable molecules which can interfere with the normal interaction of E6 and cellular proteins.

## 3.8 In conclusion

The identification of E6 and E7 as viral oncoproteins which contribute to the development of a common human cancer has provided a unique insight into the mechanisms of cervical carcinogenesis. Although additional events participating in full malignant progression remain to be fully identified, the viral nature of the disease provides potential specific targets for drug intervention or vaccination which could be used to treat at least 90% of cervical cancers.

## Acknowledgments

We would like to apologise that, due to space constraints, we have been able only to reference a small selection of the many excellent publications which have contributed to the development of this field. This work was supported in part by the National Cancer Institute, DHHS, under contract with ABL.

## References

1. **Chan, S.-Y., Delius, H., Halpern, A.L. and Bernard, H.-U.** (1995). *J. Virol.* **69:** 3074–3083.
2. **Lambert, P.F.** (1991) *J. Virol.* **65:** 3417–3420.
3. **Doorbar, J., Ely, S., Sterling, J., McLean, C. and Crawford, L.** (1991) *Nature* **352:** 824–827.
4. **Martin, P., Vass, W.C., Schiller, J.T., Lowy, D.R. and Velu, T.J.** (1989) *Cell* **59:** 21–32.
5. **Petti, L., Nilson, L.A. and DiMaio, D.** (1991) *EMBO J.* **10:** 845–855.
6. **zur Hausen, H.** (1991) *Virology* **184:** 9–13.
7. **Orth, G.** (1987). Epidermodysplasia verruciformis. in *The Papovaviridae*, Vol. 2. (eds N.P. Salzman and P.M. Howley). Plenum Publishing Corporation pp.199–243.
8. **Barr, B.B.B., McLaren, K., Smith, I.W., Benton, E.C., Bunney, M.H., Blessing, K. and Hunter, J.A.A.** (1989). *Lancet* **i:** 124–129.
9. **Pfister, H.** (1992) *Sem. Cancer Biol.* **3:** 263–271.
10. **zur Hausen, H.** (1976) *Cancer Res.* **36:** 794.
11. **Monographs, I.** (1995) in *Evaluation of Carcinogenic Risks to Humans: Human Papillomaviruses* (IACR, Lyon), Vol. 64.
12. **Dürst, M., Dzarlieva-Petrusevska, R.T., Boukamp, P., Fusenig, N.E. and Gissmann, L.** (1987) *Oncogene* **1:** 251–256.
13. **Schlegel, R., Phelps, W.C., Zhang, Y.-L. and Barbosa, M.** (1988) *EMBO J.* **7:** 3181–3187.
14. **Vousden, K.H., Doninger, J., DiPaolo, J.A. and Lowy, D.R.** (1988) *Oncogene Res.* **3:** 167–175.
15. **Hawley-Nelson, P., Vousden, K.H., Hubbert, N.L., Lowy, D.R. and Schiller, J.T.** (1989) *EMBO J.* **8:** 3905–3910.
16. **Band, V., DeCaprio, J.A., Delmolino, L., Kulesa, V. and Sager, R.** (1991) *J. Virol.* **65:** 6671–6676.
17. **McCance, D.J., Kopan, R., Fuchs, E. and Laimins, L.A.** (1988) *Proc. Natl. Acad. Sci. USA* **85:** 7169–7173.

18. Hurlin, P.J., Kaur, P., Smith, P.P., Perez-Reyes, N., Blanton, R.A. and McDougall, J.K. (1991) *Proc. Natl. Acad. Sci. USA* **88**: 571–574.
19. Phelps, W.C., Yee, C.E., Munger, K. and Howley, P.M. (1988) *Cell* **53**: 539–547.
20. Vousden, K.H. (1993) *FASEB J.* **7**: 872–879.
21. Scheffner, M., Münger, K., Byrne, J.C. and Howley, P.M. (1991) *Proc. Natl Acad. Sci. USA* **88**: 5523–5527.
22. Weinberg, R.A. (1995) *Cell* **81**: 323–330.
23. La Thangue, N.B. (1994) *Trends Biol. Sci.* **19**: 108–114.
24. Nevins, J.R. (1992) *Science* **258**: 424–429.
25. Jewers, R.J., Hildebrandt, P., Ludlow, J.W., Kell, B. and McCance, D.J. (1992) *J. Virol.* **66**: 1329–1335.
26. Defeo-Jones, D., Vuocolo, G.A., Haskell, K.M., Hanobik, M.G., Kiefer, D.M., McAvoy, E.M., Ivey-Hoyle, M., Brandsma, J.L., Oliff, A. and Jones, R.E. (1993) *J. Virol.* **67**: 716–725.
27. Boyer, S.N., Wazer, D.E. and Band, V. (1996) *Cancer Res.* **56**: 4620–4624.
28. Jones, D.L. and Münger, K. (1997) *J. Virol.* **71**: 2905–2912.
29. Hickman, E.S., Bates, S. and Vousden, K.H. (1997) *J. Virol.* **71**: 3710–3718.
30. Werness, B.A., Levine, A.J. and Howley, P.M. (1990) *Science* **248**: 76–79.
31. Scheffner, M., Werness, B.A., Huibregtse, J.M., Levine, A.J. and Howley, P.M. (1990) *Cell* **63**: 1129–1136.
32. Bates, S. and Vousden, K.H. (1996) *Current Opin. Genet. Dev.* **6**: 1–7.
33. Hunter, T. (1993) *Cell* **75**: 839–841.
34. Hollstein, M., Rice, K., Greenblatt, M.S., Soussi, T., Fuchs, R., Sørlie, T., Hovig, E., Smith-Sørensen, B., Montesano, R. and Harris, C.C. (1994) *Nuc. Acids Res.* **22**: 3551–3555.
35. Kessis, T.D., Slebos, R.J., Nelson, W.G., Kastan, M.B., Plunkett, B.S., Han, S.M., Lorincz, A.T., Hedrick, L. and Cho, K.R. (1993) *Proc. Natl Acad. Sci. USA* **90**: 3988–3992.
36. Ciechanover, A. (1994) *Cell* **79**: 13–21.
37. Scheffner, M., Huibregtse, J.M., Vierstra, R.D. and Howley, P.M. (1993) *Cell* **75**: 495–505.
38. Lane, D.P. (1992) *Nature* **358**: 15–16.
39. Crook, T., Wrede, D., Tidy, J.A., Mason, W.P., Evans, D.J. and Vousden, K.H. (1992) *Lancet* **339**: 1070–1073.
40. Klingelhutz, A.J., Foster, S.A. and McDougall, J.K. (1996) *Nature* **380**: 79–82.
41. Stoppler, H., Hartmann, D.P., Sherman, L. and Schlegel, R. (1997) *J. Biol. Chem.* **272**: 13332–13337.
42. Steller, M.A., Zou, Z., Schiller, J.T. and Baserga, R. (1996) *Cancer Res.* **56**: 5087–5091.
43. Chen, J.J., Reid, C.E., Band, V. and Androphy, E.J. (1995) *Science* **269**: 529–532.
44. Desaintes, C., Hallez, S., van Alphen, P. and Burny, A. (1992) *J. Virol.* **66**: 325–333.
45. Farthing, A.J. and Vousden, K.H. (1994) *Trends Microbiol.* **2**: 170–174.
46. Hickman, E.S., Picksley, S.M. and Vousden, K.H. (1994) *Oncogene* **9**: 2177–2181.
47. Wu, X.W. and Levine, A J. (1994) *Proc. Natl Acad. Sci. USA* **91**: 3602–3606.
48. Pan, H.C. and Griep, A.E. (1994) *Genes Dev.* **8**: 1285–1299.
49. Stoppler, M.C., Straight, S.W., Tsao, G., Schlegel, R. and McCance, D.J. (1996) *Virology* **223**: 251–254.

50. Bouvard, V., Matlashewski, G., Gu, Z.M., Storey, A. and Banks, L. (1994) *Virology* **203**: 73–80.
51. Straight, S.W., Hinkle, P.M., Jewers, R.J. and McCance, D.J. (1993) *J. Virol.* **67**: 4521–4532.
52. Goldstein, D.J., Finbow, M.E., Andresson, T., McLean, P., Smith, K., Bubb, V. and Schlegel, R. (1991) *Nature* **352**: 347–349.
53. Oelze, I., Kartenbeck, J., Crusius, K. and Alonso, A. (1995) *J. Virol.* **69**: 4489–4494.
54. Campo, M.S., Moar, M.H., Sartirana, M.L., Kennedy, I.M. and Jarrett, W.F.H. (1985) *EMBO J.* **4**: 1819–1825.
55. Jackson, M.E. and Campo, M.S. (1993) *Crit. Rev. Oncogen.* **4**: 277–291.
56. Schwarz, E., Freese, U.K., Gissmann, L., Mayer, W., Roggenbuck, B., Stremlau, A. and zur Hausen, H. (1985) *Nature* **314**: 111–114.
57. Romanczuk, H. and Howley, P.M. (1992) *Proc. Natl Acad. Sci. USA* **89**: 3159–3163.
58. May, M., Dong, X.P., Beyerfinkler, E., Stubenrauch, F., Fuchs, P.G. and Pfister, H. (1994) *EMBO J.* **13**: 1460–1466.
59. Arbeit, J. M., Howley, P. M. and Hanahan, D. (1996) *Proc. Natl Acad. Sci. USA* **93**: 2930–2935.
60. Bosch, F.X., Schwarz, E., Boukamp, P., Fusenig, N.E., Bartsch, D. and zur Hausen, H. (1990) *J. Virol.* **64**: 4743–4754.
61. Smits, P.H.M., Smits, H.L., Jebbink, M.F. and ter Schegget, J. (1990) *Virology* **176**: 158–165.
62. Crook, T. and Vousden, K.H. (1992) *EMBO J.* **11**: 3935–3940.
63. Dittmer, D., Pati, S., Zambetti, G., Chu, S., Teresky, A.K., Moore, M., Finlay, C. and Levine, A.J. (1993) *Nature Genet.* **4**: 42–46.
64. Dhanwada, K.R., Garrett, L., Smith, P., Thompson, K.D., Doster, A. and Jones, C. (1993) *J. Gen. Virol.* **74**: 955–963.
65. von Knebel Doeberitz, M., Rittmüller, C., zur Hausen, H. and Dürst, M. (1992) *Int. J. Cancer* **51**: 831–834.
66. Baer-Romero, P., Glass, S. and Rolfe, M. (1997) *Oncogene* **14**: 595–602.

## Further reading

Graham, D.A. and Herrington, C.S. (1998). The induction of chromosome abnormalities by human papillomaviruses. *Papillomavirus Report,* **9**: 1–5.

Howley, P.M. (1996) *Papillomavirinae:* The viruses and their replication. in: *Virology,* 3rd Edn. (eds B.N. Fields, D.M. Knipe, and P.M. Howley). Lippincott-Raven Press, New York, pp. 2045–2076.

Shah, K.V. and Howley, P.M. (1996) Papillomaviruses. in: *Virology,* 3rd Edn. (eds. B.N. Fields, D.M. Knipe and P.M. Howley). Lippincott-Raven Press, New York, pp. 2077–2109.

Chapter 4

# Epstein–Barr virus

## John R. Arrand

## 4.1 Introduction

Epstein–Barr virus (EBV) is a common, clinically important member of the
Herpes family of viruses. In the 30 or so years since its discovery, this virus
has attracted ever-increasing attention from medical, molecular biological,
virological and epidemiological viewpoints. It is one of the most efficient
cellular growth-transforming viruses known and yet, in the vast majority of
infected individuals, co-exists within its host completely asymptomatically.
Nevertheless, under certain circumstances its potential is unleashed and EBV
is associated with a wide spectrum of clinical conditions, many of which are
malignant. The virus has long been associated with Burkitt's lymphoma (BL)
and nasopharyngeal carcinoma (NPC) but recently has been linked to an
increasing variety of tumours of various cellular origins, many of which appear
to manifest themselves in the setting of immunosuppression, be that clinically
induced e.g. in transplant recipients or acquired via infection as in the acquired
immune deficiency syndrome.

## 4.2 Structure of EBV

The EBV particle, in common with other herpes viruses, consists of four basic
components: (i) the inner core of double-stranded DNA associated with DNA-
binding proteins; (ii) the capsid which consists of 162 capsomeres arranged in
icosahedral symmetry; (iii) an amorphous granular layer, the tegument, which
surrounds the capsid; (iv) the envelope which contains lipids and glycoproteins
involved in binding of the virion to the cell surface receptor. The structure of
the virion is shown diagrammatically in *Figure 4.1*.

  The DNA genome extracted from EBV particles is a linear, double-
stranded molecule. The prototype strain, B95-8, was obtained from a patient
with infectious mononucleosis (IM) and passaged in marmoset leucocytes. The
complete sequence of this strain has been determined and the 'standard'

*Viruses and Human Cancer*, edited by J.R. Arrand and D.R. Harper
© 1998 BIOS Scientific Publishers Ltd, Oxford

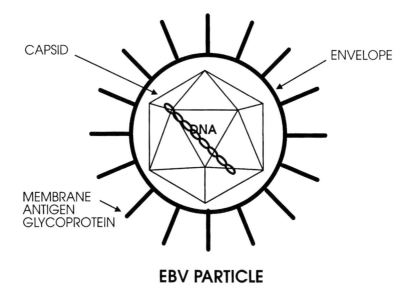

**EBV PARTICLE**

**Figure 4.1.** Diagram of herpesvirus morphology. The DNA, capsid and envelope are marked. The capsid forms an icosahedral particle as indicated by the triangles.

genome for the purpose of points of reference is deemed to be 172 281 nucleotide pairs long . However the genome is not a unique structure: it contains a variable number of terminal tandem repeats each 538 nucleotide pairs in length and a short and a long unique region of about 15 and 150 kb in size, respectively. These are separated by a variable number (5–12) of internal tandem repeats, each repeating unit being 3072 nucleotide pairs long with a non-integral number of copies. The B95-8 strain contains up to 12.6 units. This repeat region has been called IR1. In addition EBV contains other smaller repeated sequences. A region (IR2) close to the left end of the long unique region shows homology with a region (IR4) approximately 117 kb away towards the right end of the long unique region. These regions, comprising about 2 kb of DNA, consist of small tandem units. The IR2 and IR4 repeat units are 125 and 103 nucleotide pairs long, respectively. A further, distinct repeating sequence which lies within the EBNA1 coding sequence within *Bam*HI K consists of about 45 copies of the tandemly repeated sequence GGGGCAGGAGCAGGA which encodes an array of glycine and alanine. This is referred to as IR3 or the 'Gly-Ala repeat'. The organization of the genome is shown schematically in *Figure 4.2*.

Open reading frames (ORFs) within the EBV genome are named sequentially after the *Bam*HI fragment within which they begin and the direction in which they are read. Thus, for example, BZLF1 refers to *Bam*HI-**Z** leftward reading frame number **1**.

**(a)**

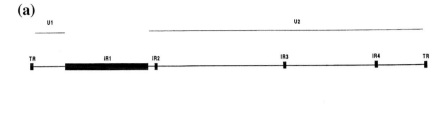

**(b)**

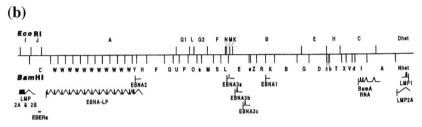

**Figure 4.2. (a)** General organization of EBV DNA. U1 and U2 are the unique sequence regions of the genome which are interspersed with the four internal repeat regions IR1–4; TR, terminal repeats. **(b)** *Eco*RI and *Bam*HI restriction endonuclease maps of EBV B95-8 DNA and the positions of the genes expressed in latency. The splicing patterns of the latent mRNAs through the coding regions are indicated. The full transcriptional patterns of the EBNA genes are more complex than shown here. See text and *Figure 4.3* for further details.

Although the EBV DNA is linear, the predominant intracellular form of the viral DNA is episomal and circular. *In situ* hybridization analysis of chromosomes from some BL-derived cell lines has provided evidence for the presence of a small number of integrated copies co-existing with the episomal form. The presence of integrants in early passage lines suggests that integration probably occurs *in vivo*. This hypothesis is supported by the finding of integrated EBV genomes in NPC biopsies [1]. Although integration of DNA has been one of the central tenets in model systems of viral carcinogenesis and seems to be involved in hepatitis B virus and human papillomavirus-(HPV)-associated oncogenesis (Sections 2.4 and 3.6.2), it is unclear as to whether it is essential in the case of EBV-associated neoplasia. Certainly in most cases, the majority of the EBV DNA within a tumour cell is episomal.

## 4.3 The viral life cycle

The stages of EBV infection were defined classically in immunological terms by the detection of antigen expression in cells in culture using naturally occurring human antibodies. These classical antigens are: (i) EBNA (EBV nuclear antigen), that is now known to consist of several distinct proteins expressed in latent infection (see Section 4.3.1); (ii) EA (early antigen), that is a complex of proteins, mainly enzymes, involved in virus replication which are expressed prior to the onset of viral DNA replication; (iii) VCA (virus capsid antigen), that comprises the components of the virion; (iv) MA (membrane antigen), the glycoproteins present on the virion envelope.

### 4.3.1 Latent infection

EBV, in its so-called latent or persistent state, maintains its genome within the cell and expresses only a limited set of genes. The combinations of these latent genes, which are expressed in different cellular/pathological situations, varies and for convenience have been classified into three latency states. In EBV-associated cancers the virus remains in one or other of these states of latency. The state now termed 'latency III' is genetically the most complex and, in order to define the full set of latent genes, it will be described first.

*Latency III.* *In vitro* infection of primary resting B cells by EBV immortalizes the cells to permanently growing lymphoblastoid cell lines (LCLs) which generally carry several copies of the viral genome in an episomal form and express only a restricted number of gene products (*Figure 4.2*). These consist of six nuclear antigens (EBNAs 1, 2, 3a, 3b and 3c, and the leader protein, EBNA-LP), three latent membrane proteins (LMPs 1, 2a and 2b) and two small RNAs known as the EBERs. In addition, a family of highly spliced RNAs which span the *Bam*HI I/A region are expressed from a promoter within *Bam*HI-I. These molecules are expressed in an antisense direction with respect to various lytic functions encoded in the same region. The function(s) of these RNAs is unknown although they do contain potential ORFs, including one, designated BARF0, which appears to encode a membrane-associated protein doublet of 30 and 35 kDa [2]. The function(s) of these molecules is not known; this pattern of latent gene expression is known as 'latency III'.

In this form of latency all the EBNA genes are part of the same transcriptional unit which is around 100 kb in length from the promoter (Cp) to the 3' end of the EBNA1 gene. A second promoter (Wp) is active immediately after infection of resting B cells by EBV but is progressively down-regulated as immortalization is established and Cp becomes dominant.

*Latency I.* Another pattern of latent gene expression, known as latency I, is found in BL (see Section 4.8.3) tumour biopsies and early passage BL cell lines *in vitro*. Here, along with the *Bam*A RNAs and the ubiquitous, abundant EBER expression, the only viral protein product is EBNA1. This selective expression of EBNA1 is the result of transcription from a different promoter (Fp) localized in the *Bam*HI F region of the genome. The Cp and Wp promoters are inactive in this situation.

*Latency II.* The final form of latency, latency II, is seen in NPC and Hodgkin's disease (HD). In this case, EBNA1 (driven by Fp) is accompanied by the LMPs, EBERs and *Bam*A RNAs.

The use of different promoters appears to be a critical factor in the regulation of EBNA gene expression and consequently the type of latency exhibited by a particular cell population. The arrangement of transcription in the three latency states is shown in *Figure 4.3*. However, it seems that, operationally useful as it may be, the latency I, II, III classification may be an oversimplification. Examination of a wider range of established B-cell lines has revealed that in addition to the exclusive use of Fp in low-passage BL lines or Cp in LCLs, some lines utilize both Fp and Cp. Such cells express EBNA2 at a lower level than that observed in LCLs and also exhibit a pattern of B-cell differentiation antigens intermediate between those seen in latency I and latency III lines. Thus, a continuum of latency states may exist for EBV-infected B cells, at least *in vitro* [3].

***Latency and the B cell.*** More recent data led Thorley-Lawson *et al.* [4] to suggest that the above nomenclature is inadequate and they have proposed an alternative scheme based on the behaviour of EBV in normal B cells. They propose three latency states: (i) the 'latency program' in which only LMP2 and possibly EBNA1 are expressed; (ii) the 'EBNA1-only program', equivalent to Latency I; (iii) the 'growth program' equivalent to Latency III. The association of these latency states with the natural history of EBV infection is discussed in Section 4.5. In the literature a variety of nomenclatures exists for the EBV

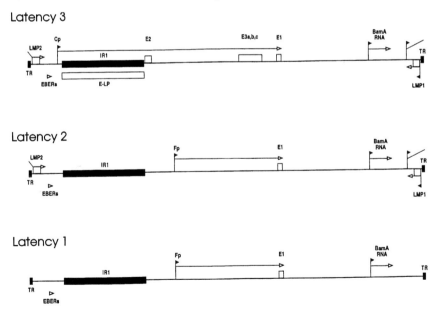

**Figure 4.3.** Schematic diagram of promoter usage and latent gene expression in the three forms of EBV latency. Promoters are shown as solid flags, RNA transcripts are horizontal arrows and protein coding regions are indicated by the open boxes. The splicing pattern of the various mRNAs are not shown, the positions of the arrows indicate only the extent of the transcriptional units.

**Table 4.1.** Nomenclature of EBV latent proteins

| | | |
|---|---|---|
| EBNA1 | | |
| EBNA2 | | |
| EBNA3a | EBNA3 | |
| EBNA3b | EBNA4 | |
| EBNA3C | EBNA6 | |
| EBNA-LP | EBNA5 | EBNA4 |
| LMP1 | | LMP |
| LMP2A | | TP1 |
| LMP2B | | TP2 |

Designations on the same horizontal line refer to the same protein.

latent genes. The various schemes are compared in *Table 4.1*.

### 4.3.2 Abortive and productive infection

Some cultures of latently infected B lymphocytes, for example Raji cells, can be induced by superinfection or by chemicals such as butyric acid or the diterpene ester 12-O-tetradecanoylphorbol-13-acetate (TPA) to synthesize EA but do not complete the full productive cycle. Such cells are termed abortively infected.

Most EBV-immortalized human B cells release no or very little virus. It has been estimated that only 0.001–0.5% of such cells produce virus. Treatment of such cell lines with chemical inducers enhances virus production approximately 10-fold.

Due to its relatively high level of production (up to 10% of the cells before induction), the most widely used cell line for the production of EBV is the B95-8 line which is a line of marmoset lymphocytes transformed by the virus.

No truly permissive, lytic host cell has as yet been identified for EBV despite extensive efforts. *In vivo*, epithelial cells may be the most active cell type involved in the production of virus particles, for example the nasopharyngeal epithelium (see Section 4.5) or the tongue in oral hairy leucoplakia (OHL) (see Section 4.8.2). *In vitro*, using epithelial cell lines transfected with the EBV receptor, it was found that following exposure to virus a high proportion of the cells were infected, expressed the EBER RNAs plus EBNA1 and that under conditions which favoured epithelial cell differentiation, up to 30% of the cells entered the productive cycle and in some instances produced VCA [5].

## 4.4 Strains of EBV

Between 80 and 90% of the total human population is infected with EBV. Therefore, there exists the potential for extensive evolutionary variability of the virus within its range worldwide. The intracellular and virion forms of EBV DNA from several sources have been examined for variation using several techniques including cross-hybridization, restriction endonuclease fragment patterns and heteroduplex analysis. All strains were shown to be very closely related. However, two of the best known strains of EBV, B95-8 and P3HR-1, are variants and both contain substantial deletions within their DNA. In B95-8 about 12.5 kb of DNA is deleted in the region of and including IR4. P3HR-1 is deleted in the EBNA2 region (see Section 4.7.1). The close inter-strain homology at the DNA level correlates well with the observation of extensive antigenic similarity on the envelopes of all strains thus examined and the fact that no distinct serotypes have been identified. The general consensus is that, excepting B95-8 and P3HR-1, all EBV DNA is very similar in structure and organization. As expected there are minor differences between isolates but the hypothesis that disease-specific subtypes exist is not favoured. Nevertheless there is evidence for a genotypic variant which occurs predominantly in NPC patients from Southern China. The variant is characterized by virtue of an additional *Bam*HI site in the *Bam*HI-F region. It was detected at higher frequency in NPC patients and among individuals with elevated EBV IgA antibodies but no apparent NPC, as compared with normal, healthy individuals or those in remission from NPC. The significance of this is not clear but may be parallel to observations on variation in the LMP gene (see below).

The overall extent of genetic variation between different isolates of EBV is uncertain. However, in spite of the overall similarity, two distinct EBV types (type A and B), often referred to as EBV-1 and EBV-2, have been defined on the basis of specific sequence variation within the EBNA2 gene encoding antigenically distinct forms of EBNA2. Further studies have revealed that such type-specific differences extend to the EBNA3 a,b,c genes and to the transcriptional units of the EBER RNAs. The two types of virus differ in biological properties in an *in vitro* transformation assay, type A being more efficient, although both types seem to contribute with equal efficiency to the pathogenesis of BL and NPC. Few comparative sequence data are available comparing A and B type viruses at other genetic loci. However it has been reported that the BZLF1 ORF and the IR1-derived coding exons for EBNA-LP of B95-8 (type A) and P3HR-1 (type B) are highly conserved; EBV MA (gp340) is highly homologous ( > 97% identity, see Section 7.5.2 and *Figure 7.7*) whilst the neighbouring genes BLLF2, BLLF3, BLRF1 and BLRF2, all of which are associated with productive infection, show even higher degrees of identity. Consequently, the pattern which is emerging shows two closely related wild-type virus strains which exhibit significant but specific divergence at several genetic loci. These variant loci appear to be confined to the latent genes, whilst proteins associated with productive infection are much more highly conserved.

Sequence analysis of the EBNA1 coding sequence within EBV genomes from a variety of sources has identified microheterogeneity which falls into a small number of subtypes [6–9]. Because of the apparent preponderance of some EBNA1 subtypes in, for example, tumour tissue it has been suggested that EBNA1 may influence the tissue tropism and life cycle of the virus [8,9]. This concept awaits verification.

Sequence analysis of the LMP1 gene from one Chinese NPC revealed considerable differences when compared with the prototype B95-8 strain and the BL-derived Raji strain. A restriction enzyme polymorphism associated with the sequence revealed that this variant was highly prevalent in southern Chinese NPC but was quite rare in similar biopsies obtained from Africa. It was suggested that the Chinese variant, which contains a 30 bp carboxyl-terminal deletion, may be more oncogenic than the prototype sequence and indeed, in an animal model system, the variant appears to be non-immunogenic [10]. This indicates a putative evasion of cytotoxic T lymphocyte (CTL) responses against NPCs which express this potential target antigen (see Section 4.6).

However, more extensive sequence comparisons from a large number of different EBV isolates, including southern Chinese NPCs and LCLs from normal, healthy carriers reveal that LMPs from all sources seem to comprise a population of variants and that no particular subtype exhibits any clear disease-association [11].

## 4.5 Natural history of EBV infection

EBV infects the human population worldwide. In western communities about 85–90% of all adults carry the virus, whereas in developing countries the infection level approaches 100% by the age of 2 years. At any given time, about 20% of virus-positive individuals shed infectious virus in saliva and this is believed to form the primary route of transmission. Recently, virus has been found to be present in breast milk from 46% of lactating women [12]. This could therefore form an alternative route of transmission to infants. Natural primary infection occurs during childhood and is generally asymptomatic. EBV, in common with other herpes viruses, establishes a persistent infection which is maintained lifelong. This persistence appears as a latent, non-productive infection of a small number (about 1 in $10^7$) of circulating lymphocytes and in some cases also as a productive infection in the oropharynx with liberation of virus into the buccal fluid. Virus has also been observed to be shed from both cervical epithelium and the male genital tract suggesting a possible sexual route of transmission in adults [13] .

It is uncertain as to which cell type provides the initial port of entry for the incoming infective virus. It could be the B lymphocyte and/or the epithelial cell. Infection of B cells is via interaction between a specific cell surface receptor, the complement receptor molecule CD21 (CR2) and the major virus envelope glycoproteins gp340/220. The interaction between EBV and the epithelial cells of the nasopharynx is not well characterized. It has been reported that some epithelial cells in culture express very low levels of CD21; alternatively, virus-infected B cells may fuse with the epithelial cell thereby delivering virus. It is well known that EBV is excreted into the saliva of the majority of healthy EBV seropositive individuals and at higher levels in patients undergoing active EBV infection. Several reports detail evidence of EBV genomes in sites surrounding the pharynx: Stensen's duct orifice, parotid glands, salivary gland epithelium and within epithelial cells of OHL (see Section 4.8.2). However, at least two other studies have detected virus in the lower respiratory tract, that is in the lung epithelium [14,15]. Collectively these data provide evidence that at least some types of epithelial cell are permissive for EBV replication. However, no site has been reproducibly demonstrated to be the major site of EBV replication within the pharynx.

The principal site of virus persistence following primary infection is also a matter of debate. It has been suggested that the basal epithelial stem cell layer maintains virus genomes in a latent state and that upon the cells' passage and differentiation through the epithelial strata, the genome becomes activated to replicate viral particles. This hypothesis is currently less favoured (see Section 4.8.2 and below) than the alternative which envisages B cells, possibly in the bone marrow [16], as being the primary site of persistence. This idea is favoured on the basis of observations that: (i) destruction of lymphoid cells (with maintenance of epithelial tissues) in EBV seropositive individuals prior to bone marrow transplantation leads to loss of the previously resident EBV infection following transplantation; (ii) prolonged acyclovir treatment for the inhibition of chronic replicative EBV infection has no effect on the number of circulating EBV-positive B cells, even though the drug eliminates virus production at epithelial sites.

In Thorley-Lawson's model [4,17] EBV is envisaged as persisting in circulating, resting B cells and supports the latency program (see Section 4.3.1.4, above), expressing only LMP2 and possibly EBNA1. However, since these resting cells do not express the co-stimulatory molecule B7, which is necessary to activate memory CTLs, the virus is invisible to the host immune response. If these resting cells encounter T-cell signalling within lymphoid tissue they may become activated to express the 'EBNA1 only' program which allows the virus genome to replicate with the cell. However, the virus is again invisible to CTL recognition by virtue of the special immune-evasion properties of EBNA1 (see Section 4.6.1). Depending on the type of signals received, these cells can return to a resting state, terminally differentiate or become apoptotic. The last two situations may lead to activation of the viral lytic cycle and production of virions. During acute infection of normal B cells, the 'growth programme' is induced. This leads to expansion of the population of infected cells, some of which may enter the resting state and maintain latency whilst the remainder are efficiently removed by CTLs. For a more detailed account of the relationship between EBV infection and the biology of B cells see [4].

## 4.6 T-cell responses to persistent infection

EBV is an extremely efficient agent for the growth transformation of B cells and yet it is carried by the vast majority of immunocompetent people in a totally asymptomatic fashion. The virus–host balance is believed to be struck in the following way. Discrete sites of virus production provide a source of virions which in turn infect B cells. These potentially growth-transformed circulating B cells exhibit a latency III phenotype and are recognized and destroyed in a human leucocyte antigen (HLA) class I-restricted context by CD8+ cytotoxic T cells. Such T cells recognize degraded forms of viral proteins which are presented at the cell surface as HLA class I–peptide complexes (see Section 7.4.3 for a more detailed description). Thus, in circulating EBV-positive B cells any or all of the latent proteins are potential sources of appropriate target peptides.

It appears that all the latent proteins, with the notable exception of EBNA1, can be targets for the CTL responses and that HLA class I type is a key determinant in the choice of target antigen: a particular allele tends to focus the response to a single viral protein, for example HLA-A11 tends to target EBNA3b. The EBNA3a,b,c family seems to be the most frequent target. Defined CTL epitopes from the EBV latent proteins are shown in *Table 4.2*.

### 4.6.1 Evasion of immune recognition

The lack of CTL responses to EBNA1 would explain the growth of EBV-associated tumours (e.g. BL, latency I, see Section 4.3.1.2) in immunocompetent individuals and also provide a framework for the concept of the maintenance of EBV latency in a population of B cells which expresses only EBNA1 as the sole EBV-encoded antigen. It has been hypothesized that the primary structure of EBNA1 does not include CTL epitopes; however, inspection of the sequence reveals several potential HLA class I epitopes. Analysis of the

**Table 4.2.** CTL epitopes from EBV latent antigens [18,19]

| Allele | Latent antigen | Epitope sequence | Type specificity |
|--------|----------------|------------------|------------------|
| DR1 | EBNA1 | TSLYNLRRGTALA | A&B |
| B18 | EBNA2 | TVFYNIPPMPL | A |
| A2 | EBNA2 | DTPLIPLTIF | A |
| A2 | EBNA3a | SVRDRLARL | A&B |
| B8 | EBNA3a | FLRGRAYGL | A |
| B8 | EBNA3a | QAKWRLQTL | A |
| ? | EBNA3a | HLAAQGMAY | A |
| B35 | EBNA3a | YPLHEQHGM | A |
| A11 | EBNA3b | IVTDFSVIK | A |
| B44 | EBNA3c | ENLLDFVRF | A&B |
| A24/B44 | EBNA3c | KEHVIQNAF | A |
| B27 | EBNA3c | RRIYDLIEL | ? |
| A2.1 | LMP2A | CLGGLLTMV | A&B |
| B27 | LMP2A | RRRWRRLTV | ? |
| A2.1 | LMP2 | LLWTLVVLL | A&B |
| A2.6 | LMP2 | LTAGFLIFL | A&B |
| A11 | LMP2 | SSCSSCPLSK | A |
| A24 | LMP2 | TYGPVFMCL | A&B |
| B40 | LMP2 | IEDPPFNSL | A&B |

All epitopes are HLA Class I restricted with the exception of the EBNA1 epitope which is HLA Class II restricted.

sequence of the EBNA1 encoding region of EBV carried within a number of spontaneous LCLs revealed that rather than all EBNA1 proteins being similar to B95-8 there exists an extensive variety of sequence microheterogeneity within potential class I-restricted epitopes of several haplotypes [6]. Experimental reactivation of memory CTL responses may therefore be critically dependent on the host/strain combination used for restimulation. Thus CTL recognition of EBNA1 may still be a determinant of the virus–host relationship during latency, with major histocompatibility complex haplotype-specific responses to particular epitopes of the protein determining which virus variants can establish persistent infection in a given individual.

A precedent for this hypothesis is found in the HLA A11-restricted epitope within EBNA3b. This epitope is conserved in most EBV type 1 isolates worldwide but is mutated with concurrent loss of antigenicity in virus isolates from southeast Asian populations where the A11 allele is highly prevalent. Epitope loss, although not to the same extent, has also been observed in the EBNA3a HLA B35 epitope in the Gambian population which has a high proportion of B35-positive individuals [20]. A similar example of epitope loss has also been observed in the case of the HPV-16 E6 protein in cervical carcinoma patients (see Section 7.4.7).

Recently an HLA class II-restricted CTL epitope has been identified within EBNA1. Interestingly this epitope appears not to be processed in B cells such that appropriate EBNA1-specific CTLs will not recognize EBNA1-expressing B lymphocytes [18]. This processing defect provides the currently favoured explanation for the immune evasion of cells exhibiting a Latency I phenotype. The defect seems to be induced by the Gly-Ala repeat (Section 4.2) since inclusion of this domain within the normally well-recognized EBNA3b protein renders cells expressing this modified antigen refractory to lysis by EBNA3b-specific CTL [21]. An additional mechanism of immune evasion (see Section 4.5, above) may be the persistence of virus in resting B cells which do not express B7.

## 4.7 Immortalization

### 4.7.1 Gene products implicated in immortalization

Identification of the immortalizing functions of EBV is clearly central to the understanding of its oncogenic potential. The lack of a fully permissive system for virus growth has been a serious obstacle to the study of EBV and for this reason there were, until recently, no genetic studies of the virus. Nevertheless, some clues were obtained as to which viral gene functions are important in the process of immortalization. Some strains of EBV such as Daudi and P3HR-1, are deleted in the region of the genome which encodes EBNA2 and EBNA-LP. These naturally occurring variants are immortalization-incompetent. Following superinfection of non-producer Raji cells with the non-immortalizing P3HR-1 strain, transforming virus could be rescued. The rescued species were recombinants between the resident and superinfecting genomes and the rescued transforming genomes had acquired the EBNA2 and EBNA-LP genes from the resident DNA. Other experiments showed that expression of EBNA2 in Rat-1 cells affected the serum requirements of the cells. These early experiments pointed to EBNA2 having a crucial role in immortalization.

Transfection of the LMP1 gene into two different rodent cell lines demonstrated that this could act as an oncogene in these cells, conferring anchorage-independence, loss of contact inhibition, reduced serum requirements and tumorigenicity in nude mice. In addition, expression of LMP1 blocked differentiation in an epithelial cell line which normally can be induced to terminally differentiate. By analogy, these results suggested a role for LMP1 in the immortalization of human B cells.

In spite of EBNA1 being the only EBV protein expressed in BL cells, classical transfection studies failed to demonstrate any immortalization function. However, the generation of EBNA1 transgenic mice led to the development of lymphomas in two of the lines of transgenics [22]. This provided the first suggestion that EBNA1 may have a direct role in immortalization. This suggestion requires further substantiation.

More recently the new EBV genetics has confirmed and extended the earlier results [23]. EBV recombinants have been constructed which either lack or have mutations in a number of genes. By these means it has been shown that EBNAs 2, 3a and 3c, EBNA-LP and LMP1 have a critical role in the transformation of B lymphocytes. The EBERs, the EBV interleukin (IL)-10 homologue (BCRF1, vIL-10) and BHRF1 which is related to the anti-apoptotic bcl-2, are all apparently dispensable as far as B-cell transformation is concerned, although more recent data indicate that the presence of exogenous vIL-10 at the time of infection significantly enhances the immortalization efficiency of B cells by both type 1 and type 2 EBV [24]. Reconstitution experiments using transfection with overlapping cosmids have shown that the '*Bam*A RNA' (*Figure 4.2*) which includes the ORF BARF0 (see Section 4.3.1.1) and which is expressed in all three latency states, is not essential for primary B-cell latent infection or transformation.

### 4.7.2 Functions of proteins involved in immortalization

The exact means by which the various latent proteins effect immortalization is not completely clear. However, some functional effects have been delineated which provide a starting point from which to attempt to unravel the mechanism of immortalization.

EBNA1 is absolutely required for the maintenance and replication of the episomal form of EBV in virus-carrying cells. It interacts with specific sequences within a region of the genome known as OriP, the origin of plasmid DNA replication, located in the *Bam*HI-C fragment. OriP and EBNA1 are the only genetic elements of the virus which are required in order that episomal replication can take place. Thus, both of these elements have at least an indirect role in immortalization by ensuring the persistence of the viral genome in the infected cell. In addition the results obtained with EBNA1 transgenic mice (see Section 4.7.1) suggest that EBNA1 may have a more substantial part to play. *In vitro* experiments show that EBNA1 can act as a transcriptional transactivator of Cp (see Section 4.3.1) and that it has properties in common with a family of RNA-binding proteins [25].

EBNA2 is expressed immediately following infection of B cells by EBV and is a transcriptional transactivator. It has been shown to up-regulate transcription of cellular genes encoding the B lymphocyte activation marker CD23, the B-lymphocyte differentiation marker CD21 and the cellular oncogene c-*fgr*. In addition, the genes for LMP1 and LMP2 are also subject to transcriptional transactivation by EBNA2. Elements within EBNA2-responsive promoters share a common core sequence which is itself not bound directly by EBNA2. Instead, a cellular protein, the human Jκ recombination signal sequence binding protein (RBP-Jκ) , interacts with EBNA2 and targets it to promoters which contain the RBP-Jκ binding sequence [26]. Interestingly, all three members of the EBNA3 family have also been shown to interact with RBP-Jκ and, at least *in vitro*, can interfere with some EBNA2-mediated effects [27]. Binding of EBNA3a or EBNA3c to RBP-Jκ prevents DNA binding whilst binding of RBP-Jκ to EBNA2 and EBNA3c is mutually exclusive. Thus, EBNA2 and the EBNA3 family may constitute a regulatory partnership in the control of RBP-Jκ-responsive genes.

RBP-Jκ has been shown to interact with mammalian Notch1 and Notch2, proteins involved in transcriptional regulation in response to the notch signalling pathway [28]. It has been suggested that EBNA2 functions by mimicking Notch signalling and that since over-expression of Notch is associated with T-cell malignancies, transcriptional activation of RBP-Jκ-responsive genes may be important in growth transformation [27,29].

LMP1 induces the transcription factor NF-κB which is a mediator of gene regulation during B-cell activation [30]. Part of this activation process is manifested by LMP1-induced expression of the B-cell activation markers CD23 and CD40 and several cellular adhesion molecules. LMP can also up-regulate expression of the cellular oncogene *bcl-2* which in turn prevents the cells from undergoing apoptosis [31]. In several forms of non-Hodgkin's lymphoma a characteristic t(14;18) translocation occurs which results in abnormal *bcl-2* expression. Expression of EBV LMP1 may provide an alternative means of inducing elevated *bcl-2*, inhibiting apoptosis and thus contributing to the early transforming event(s).

LMP1 is structurally organized into a short N-terminal cytoplasmic domain followed by six hydrophobic transmembrane domains which are followed by the highly charged cytoplasmic carboxyl terminus (CCT) (*Figure 4.4*). The CCT is 200 amino acids in length and contains two functional domains known as CTAR1 and -2 (**C**-terminal **a**ctivating **r**egion). These regions have been shown to interact with members of the cellular TRAF (tumour necrosis factor receptor associated factor) family of proteins which are involved in a signal transduction pathway leading to the activation of NF-κB. TRAFs are also targeted by tumour necrosis factor receptor (TNFR) family proteins (e.g. CD40, CD30, TNFRI, TNFRII). It is now believed that LMP1 mimics a constitutively active receptor molecule [32]. Details of the role of LMP1 and its interactions (*Figure 4.4*) in signal transduction are presented more fully by Mosialos [33].

Recent data suggest that EBNA3b, although apparently non-essential for immortalization (see Section 4.7.1), may also be able to stimulate *bcl-2* expression thereby contributing to the overall anti-apoptotic effect [34].

The first EBV genes to be expressed in the B-cell immortalization process are EBNA2 and EBNA-LP. These are followed by the rest of the EBNAs and LMP1 and finally, the EBERs. Cyclin D2 is required for resting B cells to be stimulated to progress from G0 to the active G1 phase of the cell cycle. It has been shown that EBNA2 and EBNA-LP, the first EBV genes to be expressed following infection of B cells, act in concert to activate cyclin D2 synthesis and the progression of the resting B cell into G1 [35]. In addition, EBNA2

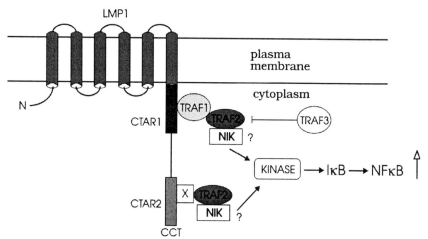

**Figure 4.4.** Schematic representation of LMP1 signalling complexes at the plasma membrane (redrawn from Mosialos, 1997, Epstein-Barr Virus Report, Volume 4 with permission from Leeds Medical Information). The six transmembrane domains are represented as cylinders and the short cytoplasmic amino-terminal and long carboxyl-terminal cytoplasmic domains are indicated by N and CCT, respectively. The two NF-κB-activating domains within the CCT are shown as CTAR1 and CTAR2. CTAR1 binds to TRAF1, TRAF2 and TRAF3. TRAF1–TRAF2 heterodimers bind constitutively to CTAR1 and probably recruit other cellular factors that propagate a signal transduction cascade. The TRAF2–associated kinase NIK may participate in this pathway by activating a protein kinase cascade that leads to IκB phosphorylation and degradation and ultimately activation of NF-κB. TRAF3 competes with TRAF1 and TRAF2 for binding to CTAR1 and it may act to down-regulate the NF-κB-activating signal that is generated by TRAF1–TRAF2 heterodimers. CTAR2 is located within the carboxyl-terminal 35 amino acids. The cellular factor(s) (X) that mediate CTAR2 signalling are currently unknown, however, several lines of evidence suggest that TRAF2 or a related protein mediates NF-κB activation from CTAR2.

confers resistance to the antiproliferative effect of alpha interferon [36] (compare with HHV-8, see Section 5.7).

Binding of gp340/220 to CD21 during infection of B cells (see Section 4.5) induces IL-6 which can act as an autocrine growth factor and can also inhibit the immune system allowing for the promotion of B-cell tumours by impairing lymphokine-activated killer cells [37]. Again, there are parallels with HHV-8 (see Section 5.9).

## 4.8 Clinical significance

In spite of the virus' usual state of benign persistence, it is nevertheless associated with a variety of clinical conditions, many of which are malignant. These include BL, NPC, lymphomas in organ transplant patients following immunosuppressive therapy, an inherited condition known as X-linked lymphoproliferative syndrome or Duncan's disease in which afflicted individuals fail to mount an effective immune response to EBV with eventually fatal consequences, Hodgkins disease (HD), gastric cancer and a variety of AIDS-associated complications including lymphoma and OHL.

### 4.8.1 Infectious mononucleosis

In developed countries primary infection is often delayed for several years. Following first time infection during adolescence or young adulthood, clinical IM develops in about half of the instances. It has been surmised that the reason for the development of IM in adolescents as compared with asymptomatic primary infection in infants is related to the size of the dose of incoming, orally transmitted virus. Clearly salivary exchange between amorous teenagers is much higher than that from adult to infant or child to child. In the USA alone, it is estimated that there are about 100 000 new cases of IM per year. This disease resembles a self-limited leukaemia in that the abnormal proliferation of lymphocytes spontaneously subsides. Although the disease is not generally life-threatening it is a cause of significant morbidity.

### 4.8.2 Oral hairy leukoplakia

OHL is an AIDS-associated lesion of the epithelial cells of the tongue. It presents as raised white areas with a rough ('hairy') appearance. The cells of the outermost, differentiated layers of the affected epithelium contain EBV particles and it has been suggested that OHL represents an exaggerated form of the normal epithelial cell infection by EBV (i.e. the site of productive infection) [38]. The degree of genome activation correlates with the extent of epithelial cell differentiation, that is the fully permissive cells are the most differentiated. By analogy with HPV it was anticipated that the basal cells of the epithelium would carry latent virus. This appears not to be the case: the virus is absent from the lower layers suggesting that cycles of virus release and cellular infection take place only in the upper layers. Thus, in this situation epithelial cells do not appear to be a site of EBV persistence (see Section 4.5).

### 4.8.3 Burkitt's lymphoma

BL (see also Section 1.3) is perhaps the classic virus-associated human cancer [39]. The tumour occurs predominantly in children and is endemic in the malarial belts of Africa (*Figure 4.5*) where it affects about 10 in every 100 000 children per year, and in New Guinea. Studies in Uganda show that around 70% of the cases of BL occur in the 5–9-year-old age group. The incidence of the tumour in these areas is influenced by temperature and rainfall and the climate-dependent co-factor appears to be hyperendemic malaria. Outside the endemic areas BL occurs worldwide at a low frequency (sporadic BL) and this form of the disease is generally accepted to be EBV-negative (but see below). The primary molecular abnormality in both the EBV-positive (endemic) and EBV-negative (sporadic) forms of BL is specific chromosomal translocations which result in the enhanced expression of the cellular oncogene c-*myc* from an immunoglobulin locus. This has led to the hypothesis that EBV is itself a co-factor and not a cause in the development of BL by virtue of its role in expanding the pre-B-cell population thereby increasing the chances of the critical translocation occurring (see [40] for recent review). Against this theory must be set the intriguing recent observations on the BL cell line Akata. During propagation *in vitro* it was observed that the viral genome was being lost from some of the cells. Isolation of EBV-positive and EBV-negative clones from the

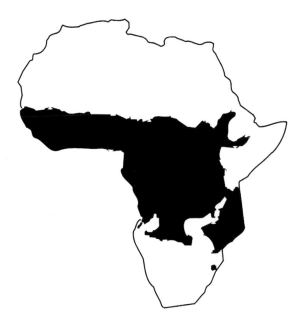

**Figure 4.5.** Map of Africa indicating (in black), the high-incidence area of endemic Burkitt's lymphoma.

same population revealed that along with the viral genome, the EBV-negative cells had lost their malignant potential as assayed by growth in low serum, anchorage independence in soft agar and tumorigenicity in nude mice [41]. These observations serve to underline the role of EBV as an oncogenic agent in humans.

Recently, partial EBV genomes have been found in some cases of sporadic BL. It has been suggested that this may represent viral DNA rearrangement and loss during malignant progression and that EBV may have an initiating role in the genesis of these tumours [42]. The various lines of evidence implicating EBV as playing a part in the aetiology of endemic BL have been set out in several texts (see, for example [43]). A striking piece of evidence for EBV's role in BL comes from a World Health Organisation (WHO) prospective study initiated in 1972 in Uganda. In this work 42 000 children were followed serologically for the level of anti-EBV IgG antibody. The study demonstrated that children destined to develop endemic BL show unusually high titres of antibodies against VCA compared with controls. It was calculated that children with a VCA titre two doubling dilutions or more above controls had a 30-fold greater risk of developing endemic BL [44]. Epstein pointed out that such a risk factor is greater than that accepted as establishing an aetiological relationship between smoking and lung cancer.

As mentioned above (Section 4.3.1.2) BL cells have a latency I phenotype. This presumably enables escape from EBV-specific immune surveillance by virtue of the lack of appropriate specific CTL targets (see Section 4.6).

BL is perhaps the fastest-growing tumour in man. It has a potential doubling time of around 24 h and a growth fraction (proportion of proliferating cells) approaching 100%. Probably because of this extremely rapid cellular proliferation the tumour responds particularly well to chemotherapy which is the treatment of choice. It is one of the very few tumours which is potentially curable solely by drugs and is often treated successfully.

### 4.8.4 Immunoblastic lymphoma

A significant complication in the management of immunocompromised patients such as those suffering from AIDS or recipients of kidney, heart, liver, thymus or allogeneic bone marrow transplants is the development of EBV-driven immunoblastic lymphomas [45,46]. Lymph nodes and other tissues such as the central nervous system may become infiltrated with mono-, oligo-, or polyclonal, EBV genome-positive, immature B lymphocytes. Analysis of the viral gene expression pattern in these lesions reveals a latency III phenotype reminiscent of that found in LCLs established by *in vitro* infection. The implication here is that these lesions are primarily driven by EBV. Such lymphomas may regress following easing of immunosuppression in transplant recipients presumably due to restoration of EBV-specific CTL control acting on the spectrum of latent proteins expressed by the tumour cells. There is no evidence of any consistent secondary genetic change in the development of these tumours,

EBV immortalization in the setting of immune suppression seems to be sufficient.

Whilst the majority of central nervous system lymphomas in AIDS patients appear to follow the pattern outlined above, other systemic, AIDS-related lesions are more heterogeneous and in some cases exhibit a latency II pattern of expression. The basis of this diversity in the AIDS group is currently unclear.

Although reduction of immunosuppression may result in remission of disease, post-transplant immunoblastic lymphomas are often refractory to treatment. The tumour cells are usually of donor origin and two recent trials have investigated the utility of reinfusion of donor T cells to combat lymphoproliferation [47,48]. The first study [47] used unseparated leucocytes from EBV-seropositive donors whereas in the second trial EBV-specific CTL were prepared from donors. In both trials some success was achieved in combatting EBV-related lymphoproliferation. This form of adoptive transfer therapy may become one of the most effective modes of treatment for the future.

### 4.8.5 Hodgkin's lymphoma

Whilst BL and NPC are geographically restricted in their principal high incidence areas, the lymphoma known as Hodgkin's disease is much more widespread and has an incidence of 2–4 per 100 000 in western Europe and the USA. Recent data suggest an involvement of EBV in a proportion of cases of this common tumour [49,50].

Case–control studies have shown that patients with HD have elevated anti-EBV antibody titres and in addition it has been found that altered EBV serology precedes the onset of the disease. Furthermore, individuals who have had clinical IM show an increased predisposition to subsequent development of HD.

HD is an unusual cancer in that the malignant cells of the tumour mass, the Reed–Sternberg (RS) cells, constitute only a small proportion of the total. The different histological subtypes of HD are distinguished on the basis of the normal cell infiltrate. The derivation of the RS cells is unclear in that they appear to be of lymphoid origin but cannot be assigned unequivocally as belonging to either the B or T lineage. For a more detailed discussion of RS cells see Stein *et al.* [51].

Southern blot analysis of DNA extracted from HD lesions revealed the presence of EBV DNA in around 20% of cases. Analysis of the terminal fragments of the viral genome indicated monoclonality. *In situ* hybridization studies have demonstrated that the virus genome is present in the RS cells in up to 50% of cases. Taken with the monoclonality data this suggests that the virus must have entered the RS cells prior to clonal expansion and therefore is suggestive of a role of the virus in the early development of the tumour.

*In situ* hybridization of the abundant EBER RNAs revealed that in addition to the RS cells, EBV could also be detected in a proportion of small lymphocytes within the tumour. Immunocytochemical staining revealed expression of LMP1 but not EBNA2 in the RS cells whereas the lymphocytes were LMP1-negative. Similar EBER-positive, LMP1-negative lymphocytes can be found in lymph nodes from normal, healthy, seropositive individuals. Thus, EBV gene expression in the malignant RS cells of HD is similar to that found in NPC, that is latency II. EBV appears at different frequency in the various histological subtypes of HD. In mixed cellularity HD around 70% of cases are positive; in nodular sclerosing HD the level is about 40% whereas in lymphocyte predominant disease the rate is only around 14%. However, LMP1 itself can be a target for CTLs in normal, healthy individuals (see Section 4.6). This suggests that in HD (and NPC) patients there are immunological deficiencies which allow the tumour cells to evade immune surveillance and proliferate.

### 4.8.6 X-Linked lymphoproliferative syndrome

The X-linked lymphoproliferative syndrome (XLP, Duncan's Syndrome) [52] is a relatively rare condition which occurs in males who carry a defect on the X chromosome at the lymphoproliferative control locus. Males with XLP are completely normal in many immune functions but are deficient in their response to EBV. These defects include reduced antibody titres against EA and VCA and a complete absence of any EBNA response. Patients with XLP do not succumb to infectious agents which do not infect the immune system itself, including other human herpes viruses, herpes simplex virus, cytomegalovirus, and varicella zoster virus, whereas EBV (which infects within the immune system) is not tolerated. Infection leads to fatal IM in about 65% of cases. A defect in T-cell surveillance appears to allow the EBV-driven abnormal proliferation which frequently results in liver failure due to lymphoid infiltration. About 35% of cases develop malignant lymphoma.

### 4.8.7 T-cell lymphomas

EBV is commonly referred to as being B lymphotropic. It was therefore surprising when the virus was found in T lymphoma cells [53]. Even though it had been known for some time that certain T cells possess the EBV receptor, attempts at obtaining viral infection of such cells *in vitro* had proved uniformly negative. This observation has been confirmed in an increasing number of instances and in a variety of T-cell lesions. In some studies the rate of EBV association was quite high, for example 62% in an examination of peripheral T-cell lymphomas in China. A complicating factor in some cases is that the EBV genome appears in only a proportion of the tumour cells thus suggesting that EBV infection may be a secondary event within an already established tumour; nevertheless, this may confer a growth advantage which ultimately leads to an EBV-positive, clonal mass.

An interesting association between two human tumour viruses has been observed in certain cases of human T-cell leukaemia virus (HTLV-I)-associated adult T-cell leukaemia/lymphoma (for a more detailed discussion of this condition see Chapter 6). One study [54] found that 17% of such lesions contained EBV in addition to HTLV-I thus raising the possibility of synergism between genes from two oncogenic viruses present in the same cell contributing to the development of the disease. The EBV-positive cells expressed both EBNA2 and LMP1. Similar synergistic effects have been postulated for HTLV-I and HPV or hepatitis C virus (see Section 6.3.1.1).

### 4.8.8 Nasopharyngeal carcinoma

EBV is implicated in the aetiology of NPC, a malignant epithelial tumour of the post-nasal space. NPC is classified into three histopathological types as designated by the World Health Organization: class I, squamous cell carcinoma (differentiated); class II, non-keratinized carcinoma (partially differentiated); class III, poorly/undifferentiated. For details of this classification system and a wider discussion of NPC, see [55].

The incidence of NPC varies widely with geographic location, age and race. It occurs mainly (15–30 cases per 100 000 population) in Hong Kong and the southern provinces of China (*Figure 4.6*) where, in some areas, such as

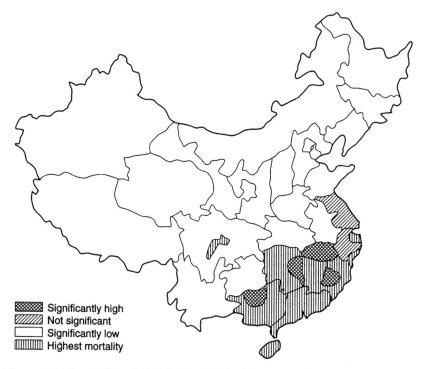

Significantly high
Not significant
Significantly low
Highest mortality

**Figure 4.6.** Map of China indicating the high incidence areas for NPC. Re-drawn from Fang, 1986, Geographica Medica, volume 16, with permission of Akadémiai Kiadó [56].

parts of the Provinces of Guangdong and Guangxi, it is the most prevalent malignancy of males and the second most common of women. Given the large population density of China, this high incidence makes NPC a very significant cancer in global numerical terms. Although rare throughout the rest of the world, small areas of high frequency are found in Alaska, Greenland and parts of central and north Africa. In contrast to BL, NPC is a disease of older age groups. Statistics from Hong Kong show a peak incidence at 50–60 years of age (*Figure 4.7*).

The association between EBV and NPC was first revealed in serological

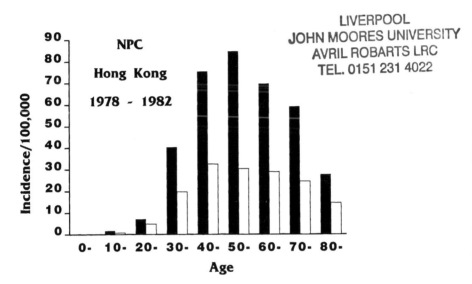

**Figure 4.7.** Age and sex distribution and incidence of NPC in Hong Kong. The solid and open bars show cases in males and females, respectively. The data are taken from [57].

studies. A characteristic pattern of responses to EBV antigens has been confirmed for different geographical populations whether they exhibit high, intermediate or low incidence of disease. Patients with type II or III NPC show elevated titres of antibodies to VCA, diffuse components of the early antigen complex (EA–D) and to the virus-encoded DNase and thymidine kinase enzymes [58]. The most striking feature of this EBV-related serology is a significant IgA response which may be detected at a 10-fold higher concentration than in control samples. Such an IgA response has not been noted in other EBV-associated diseases. The value of EBV serological markers in the evaluation (diagnosis/prognosis) of NPC patients should not be underestimated; disease progression correlates with a rise in EBV antibody titres, while tumour resection is followed by a decline in these levels. Moreover, rises in EA titre precede the onset of NPC by 2–3 years [59].

The link between EBV and both BL and NPC has been reinforced by data demonstrating the presence of EBV nucleic acids and proteins in biopsies from the two types of tumour. EBV DNA is detected consistently in class II or III NPC and in the vast majority of endemic African BL cases. Well-differentiated NPC (WHO class I) is generally thought not to have a special association with EBV. However, some workers [60] have found EBV DNA in class I biopsies, suggesting that all histological subtypes of NPC may contain EBV DNA. However this conclusion remains controversial [61].

Examination of latent protein expression in NPC biopsies revealed the ubiquitous EBNA1 and EBER expression and detectable amounts of LMP1 in around 50% of the samples (i.e. a latency I/II phenotype). Again this suggests evasion of immunological surveillance by non-expression of important target epitopes.

Recent studies using *in situ* hybridization for the detection of EBV nucleic acids in tissue sections have detected the presence of the virus in tumour cells within carcinoma *in situ* (CIS) lesions [62]. Whilst some of these CIS lesions had progressed to the microinvasive stage, some had not. Thus, EBV appears to be involved in the very early stages of development of an NPC lesion. However, it is not yet clear whether the virus plays a part in the initiation of the tumour or whether infection of a candidate tumour cell by the virus confers a selective growth advantage such that EBV-positive tumour cells become the dominant population as the lesion progresses.

The early symptoms of NPC are very often vague and tend to be ignored by the patient. Consequently initial presentation is frequently delayed until the tumour is at a relatively advanced stage. NPC is a rapidly growing tumour with a tendency to metastasize early to the lymph nodes of the neck and also to distant sites such as bone, liver and lung. The primary tumour is radiosensitive and radiotherapy is the definitive treatment. However, 5-year survival rates are, at best, around 40%.

### 4.8.9 Gastric carcinoma

Recent studies have revealed an apparent association of EBV with a proportion of gastric carcinomas [63]. This cancer is relatively frequent and is of particular importance in Japan where it is the most common cancer (approximately 95 000 new cases per annum). Studies using *in situ* hybridization and antibody staining reveal the presence of EBV in about 7% of the total cases in Japanese patients. Studies in a series of North American patients indicated a frequency of around 16% whilst in the UK the figure is around 4%. Interestingly, as in NPC, the virus is found in virtually all cases of undifferentiated gastric carcinomas but is rare in more differentiated types. EBV genomes are present in all the malignant carcinoma cells but not in infiltrating lymphocytes or in normal mucosa. The virus also appears to be involved in metastatic lymph nodes. Analysis of the terminal fragments of the viral DNA within the tumour cells indicates monoclonality. Some reports observe a latency II pattern of expression whilst others claim a novel form of latent gene expression, namely EBNA1 and LMP2a.

### 4.8.10 Smooth muscle tumours

Recent findings have revealed the presence of EBV genomes in smooth muscle tumours occurring in children and young people with immunosuppression due to either AIDS or therapy following organ transplantation [64,65]. The viral genomes within the tumour cells were clonal, implying a causal relationship between EBV infection and the subsequent proliferation of the muscle cells. Studies on viral gene expression in the tumours from the transplant patients showed that EBNA2 was expressed but LMP appeared to be absent. Whether this represents a further class of EBV latent gene expression awaits further experimental clarification.

## 4.9 Co-factors

With the probable exception of the immunoblastic lymphomas (see Section 4.8.4) the environmental and genetic co-factors involved in many EBV-associated malignancies are consistent with EBV infection being one stage in a multi-step carcinogenesis process (see also Sections 1.3, 2.7, 3.6). It has been shown that around 30% of BL biopsies contain mutations within the p53 gene and that many of these mutations have the ability to reduce the normal suppressive effect of p53 on DNA synthesis. It is thought likely that mutation of p53 may be an important step in the development of some BL tumours [40]. On the contrary, immunoblastic lymphoma and NPC rarely contain mutant p53 [66,67].

Epidemiological studies support the significance of genetic co-factors, possibly HLA type and/or a predisposition gene, in the aetiology of NPC [68], in contrast to BL where the high endemic frequency of certain regions is not correlated with ethnic groups but to climate-determined factors (see Section 4.8.3).

In the case of NPC a favoured hypothesis is that elevated levels of certain nitrosamines in the diet act in concert with EBV to generate the tumour. Such nitrosamines have been found in dried, salted fish which is a traditional ethnic food among Chinese in the high-risk regions. Rats which were fed on such fish developed more tumours than controls. Similar nitrosamines have also been detected in traditional foods from two other high risk areas, Greenland and Tunisia [69,70].

A second potential source of co-factors is found in the indigenous plant life of southern China. Certain species of the genus *Croton*, *Euphorbia* and some others have been found to contain compounds which either enhance the transforming efficiency of EBV *in vitro* or function as activators of viral gene expression in much the same way as TPA. These plants grow by rivers and near roads and thus the active compounds may be ingested in drinking water or inhaled as dust [71]. However, similar plants are also found in areas where the frequency of NPC is low.

## 4.10 EBV as a human tumour virus

As alluded to in some of the preceding sections, it is very difficult to obtain absolute proof of a causal relationship between infection by a virus and development of a human cancer. In 1971, Henle [72] modified Koch's postulates (see Section 1.5) and proposed criteria to be fulfilled by a potential tumour virus in order for it to be accepted as being oncogenic in man. These criteria are:

(i)    detection of virus, virus-determined antigens or virus-related nucleic acids in human tumours;
(ii)   induction of tumours in non-human primates by inoculation of virus;
(iii)  transformation of normal cells by virus *in vitro;*
(iv)   demonstration of antibodies to virus-related antigens at higher frequencies and/or higher titres in patients with given malignancies than in healthy individuals or patients with other tumours.

All of these criteria have been fulfilled by EBV:

(i)    EBV DNA, RNA and latent proteins have been found in the tumours discussed above but not in many other tumours;
(ii)   inoculation of EBV into cottontop tamarins results in the development of malignant lymphoproliferative disease (see Chapter 7);
(iii)  virus with transforming ability for human B lymphocytes is readily recovered from throat washings of individuals with IM. The virally transformed cells contain the EBV genome and express the latent proteins;
(iv)   all Chinese patients with NPC as well as all African patients with BL have anti-EBV antibodies at a higher level than controls.

## 4.11 Conclusions

Clearly EBV is associated with a wide variety of human malignancies. In most cases the indications are that the virus is necessary but not sufficient for the development of the cancer. In the case of immunoblastic lymphomas EBV alone may be the culprit. Final proof of the indispensability of EBV (or any other virus) as an oncogenic agent in human neoplasia probably rests in the demonstration of prevention of the appropriate tumour by vaccination against the virus. The development of such vaccines is described in Chapter 7.

## References

1. **Kripalani-Joshi, S. and Law, H.Y.** (1994) *Int. J. Cancer* **56:** 187–192.
2. **Fries, K.L., Sculley, T.B., Webster-Cyriaque, J., Rajadurai, P., Sadler, R.H. and Raab-Traub, N.** (1997) *J. Virol.* **71:** 2765–2771.

3. Taylor, K.A., Wetzel, S., Lyles, D.S. and Pollok, B.A. (1994) *J. Virol.* **68:** 6421–6431.
4. Thorley-Lawson, D.A., Miyashita, E.M. and Khan, G. (1996) *Trends Microbiol.* **4:** 204–208.
5. Li, Q-X., Young, L.S., Niedobitek, G., Dawson, C.W., Birkenbach, M., Wang, F. and Rickinson, A.B. (1992) *Nature* **356:** 347–350.
6. Wrightham, M.N., Stewart, J.P., Janjua, N.J., Pepper, S. de V., Sample, C., Rooney, C.M. and Arrand, J.R. (1995) *Virology* **208:** 521–530.
7. Snudden, D.K., Smith, P.R., Lai, D., Ng, M.-H. and Griffin, B.E. (1995) *Oncogene* **10:** 1545–1552.
8. Bhatia, K., Raj, A., Gutiérrez, M.I., Judde, J.-G., Spangler, G., Venkatesh, H. and Magrath, I.T. (1996) *Oncogene* **13:** 177–181.
9. Gutiérrez, M.I., Raj, A., Spangler, G., Sharmer, A., Hussain, A., Judde, J.-G., Tsao, S.W., Yuen, P.W., Joab, I., Magrath, I.T. and Bhatia, K. (1997) *J. Gen. Virol.* **78:** 1663–1670.
10. Trivedi, P., Hu, L-F., Chen, F., Christensson, B., Masucci, M.G., Klein, G. and Winberg, G. (1994) *Eur. J. Cancer* **30A:** 84–88.
11. Sandvej, K., Gratama, J.W., Munch, M., Zhou, X.G., Bolhuis, R.L., Andresen, B.S., Gregersen, N. and Hamilton–Dutoit, S. (1997) *Blood* **90:** 323–330.
12. Junker, A.K., Thomas, E.E., Radcliffe, A., Forsyth, R.B., Davidson, A.G.F. and Rymo, L. (1991) *Am. J. Med. Sci.* **302:** 220–223.
13. Israele, V., Shirley, P. and Sixbey, J.W. (1991) *J. Infect. Dis.* **163:** 1341–1343.
14. Lung, M.L., Lam, W.K., So, S.Y., Lam, W.P., Chan, K.H. and Ng, M.H. (1985) *Lancet* **i:** 889–892.
15. Egan, J.J., Stewart, J.P., Hasleton, P.S., Arrand, J.R., Carroll, K.B. and Woodcock, A.A. (1995) *Thorax* **50:** 1234–1239.
16. Gratama, J.W., Oosterveer, M.A.P., Zwaan, F.E., Lepoutre, J., Klein, G. and Ernberg, I. (1988) *Proc. Natl. Acad. Sci. USA* **85:** 8693–8696.
17. Miyashita, E.M., Yang, B., Babcock, G.J. and Thorley–Lawson, D.A. (1997) *J. Virol.* **71:** 4882–4891.
18. Moss, D.J., Burrows, S.R., Suhrbier, A. and Khanna, R. (1994) in *Vaccines Against Virally Induced Cancers*. Ciba Foundation Symposium **187:** John Wiley & Sons, Chichester. pp. 4–13.
19. Lee, S.P., Tierney, R.J., Thomas, W.J., Brooks, J.M. and Rickinson, A.B. (1997) *J. Immunol.* **158:** 3325–3334.
20. Lee, S.P., Morgan, S., Skinner, J., Thomas, W.A., Rowland-Jones, S., Sutton, J., Khanna, R., Whittle, H.C. and Rickinson, A.B. (1995) *Eur. J. Immunol.* **25:** 102–110.
21. Levitskaya, J., Coram, M., Levitsky, V., Steigerwald-Mullen, P.M., Klein, G., Kurilla, M.G. and Masucci, M.G. (1995) *Nature* **375:** 685–688.
22. Wilson, J.B, Bell, J.L. and Levine, A.J. (1996) *EMBO J.* **15:** 3117–3126.
23. Kieff, E., Izumi, K., Kaye, K., Longnecker, R., Mannick, J., Miller, C., Robertson, E., Swaminathan, S., Tomkinson, B., Tung, X. and Yalamanchili, R. (1994) in *Viruses and Cancer.* (eds A. Minson, J. Neil and M. McCrae). Cambridge University Press, Cambridge, pp. 123–147.
24. Stuart, A.D., Stewart, J.P., Arrand, J.R. and Mackett, M. (1995) *Oncogene* **11:** 1711–1719.
25. Snudden, D.K., Hearing, J., Smith, P.R., Grässer, F.A. and Griffin, B.E. (1994) *EMBO J.* **13:** 4840–4847.

26. Waltzer, L., Logeat, F., Brou, C., Israel, A., Sergeant, A. and Manet, E. (1994) *EMBO J.* **13**: 5633–5638.
27. Robertson, E.S., Lin, J. and Kieff, E. (1996) *J. Virol.* **70**: 3068–3074.
28. Artavanis–Tsakonas, S., Matsuno, K. and Fortini, M.E. (1995) *Science* **268**: 225–232.
29. Hsieh, J.J-D, Nofziger, D.E., Weinmaster, G. and Hayward, S.D. (1997) *J. Virol.* **71**: 1938–1945.
30. Klaman, L.D. and Thorley–Lawson, D.A. (1995) *J. Virol.* **69**: 871–881.
31. Henderson, S., Rowe, M., Gregory, C., Croom-Carter, D., Wang, F., Longnecker, R., Kieff, E. and Rickinson, A. (1991) *Cell* **65**: 1107–1115.
32. Gires, O., Zimber-Strobl, U., Gonnella, R., Ueffing, M., Marschall, G., Zeidler, R., Pich, D. and Hammerschmidt, W. (1997) *EMBO J.* **16**: 6131–6140.
33. Mosialos, G. (1997) *Epstein–Barr Virus Report* **4**: 121–126.
34. Silins, S. and Sculley, T.B. (1995) *Int. J. Cancer* **60**: 65–72.
35. Sinclair, A.J., Palmero, I., Peters, G. and Farrell, P.J. (1994) *EMBO J.* **13**: 3321–3328.
36. Aman, P. and von Gabain, A. (1990) *EMBO J.* **9**: 147–152.
37. Tanner, J.E. and Alfieri, C. (1996) *Leuk. Lymphoma* **21**: 379–390.
38. Greenspan J.S., Greenspan D., Lennette E.T., Abrams D.I., Conant M.A., Petersen, V., and Freese U.K. (1985) *N. Engl. J. Med.* **313**: 1564–1571.
39. Burkitt, D. (1983) *Cancer* **51**: 1777–1786.
40. Farrell, P.J. and Sinclair, A.J. (1994) in *Viruses and Cancer.* (eds A. Minson, J. Neil and M. McCrae). Cambridge University Press, Cambridge, 1994. pp. 101–121.
41. Shimizu, N., Tanabe-Tochikura, A., Kuroiwa, Y. and Takada, K. (1994) *J. Virol.* **68**: 6069–6073.
42. Razzouk, B.I., Srinivas, S., Sample, C.E., Singh, V. and Sixbey, J.W. (1996) *J. Infect. Dis.* **173**: 529–535.
43. Epstein, M.A. and Achong, B.G. (eds) (1979) *The Epstein–Barr Virus.* Springer-Verlag, Berlin, Heidelberg, New York.
44. de Thé, G., Geser, A., Day, N.E., *et al.* (1978) *Nature* **274**: 756–761.
45. MacMahon, E.M.E., Glass, J.D., Hayward, S.D., Mann, R.B., Becker, P.S., Charache, P., McArthur, J.C. and Ambinder, R.F. (1991) *Lancet* **338**: 969–973.
46. Randhawa, P.S., Jaffe, R., Demetris, A.J., Nalesnik, M., Starzl, T.E., Chen, Y.Y. and Weiss, L.M. (1992) *New Engl. J. Med.* **327**: 1710–1714.
47. Papadopoulos, E.B., Ladanyi, M., Emanuel, D., *et al.* (1994). *New Engl. J. Med.* **330**: 1185–1191.
48. Rooney, C.M., Smith, C.A., Ng, C.Y.C., Loftin, S., Li., C., Krance, R.A., Brenner, M.K. and Heslop, H.E. (1995) *Lancet* **345**: 9–13.
49. Herbst, H., Steinbrecher, E., Niedobitek, G., Young, L.S., Brooks, L., Müller-Lantzch, N. and Stein, H. (1992) *Blood* **80**: 484–491.
50. Deacon, E.M., Pallesen, G., Niedobitek, G., Crocker, J., Brooks, L., Rickinson, A.B. and Young, L.S. (1993) *J. Exp. Med.* **177**: 339–349.
51. Stein, H., Herbst, H., Anagnostopoulos, I., Niedobitek, G., Dallenbach, F. and Kratzsch, H.-C. (1991) *Ann. Oncol.* **2 (Suppl. 2)**: 33–38.
52. Purtilo, D.T. (1985) *Biomed. Pharmacother.* **39**: 52–58.
53. Chen, C.-L., Sadler, R.H., Walling, D.M., Su, I.-J., Hsieh, H.-C. and Raab-Traub, N. (1993) *J. Virol.* **67**: 6303–6308.

54. Tokunaga, M., Imai, S., Uemura, Y., Tokudome, T., Osato, T. and Sato, E. (1993) *Am. J. Pathol.* **143**: 1263–1269.
55. Simons, M.J. and Shanmugaratnam, K. (1982. *The Biology of Nasopharyngeal Carcinoma.* UICC Technical Report, **71**: UICC, Geneva.
56. Fang, R. (1986) *Geogr. Med.* **16**: 11–26.
57. Muir, C., Waterhouse, J., Mack, T., Powell, J. and Whelan, S. (eds) (1987) *Cancer Incidence in Five Continents.* Vol. V. IARC Scientific Publication 88. International Agency for Research on Cancer, Lyon.
58. Littler, E., Baylis, S.A., Zeng, Y., Conway, M.J., Mackett, M. and Arrand, J.R. (1991) *Lancet* **337**: 685–689.
59. de Thé, G. and Zeng, Y. (1986) in *The Epstein–Barr Virus: Recent Advances.* (eds M.A. Epstein and B.G. Achong) William Heinemann, London, pp. 237–249.
60. Raab-Traub, N., Flynn, K., Pearson, G., Huang, A., Levine, P., Lanier, A. and Pagano, J.S. (1987) *Int. J. Cancer* **39**: 25–29.
61. Niedobitek, G., Hansmann, M.L., Herbst, H., *et al.* (1991) *J. Pathol.* **165**: 17–24.
62. Yeung, W.M., Zong, Y.S., Chiu, C.T., Chan, K.H., Sham, J.S.T., Choy, D.T.K. and Ng, M.H. (1993) *Int. J. Cancer,* **53**: 746–750.
63. Imai, S., Koizumi, S., Sugiura, M., Tokunaga, M., Uemura, Y., Yamamoto, N., Tanaka, S., Sato, E. and Osato, T. (1994) *Proc. Natl Acad. Sci. USA* **91**: 9131–9135.
64. McClain, K.L., Leach, C.T., Jenson, H.B., Joshi, V.V., Pollock, B.H., Parmley, R.T., DiCarlo, F.J., Chadwick, E.G. and Murphy, S.B. (1995) *New Engl. J. Med.* **332**: 12–18.
65. Lee, E.S., Locker, J., Nalesnik, M., Reyes, J., Jaffe, R., Alashari, M., Nour, B., Tzakis, A. and Dickman, P.S. (1995) *New Engl. J. Med.* **332**: 19–25.
66. Edwards, R.H. and Raab-Traub, N. (1994) *J. Virol.* **68**: 1309–1315.
67. Spruck, C.H., Tsai, Y.C., Huang, D.P., Yang, A.S., Rideout, W.M., Gonzalez–Zulueta, M., Choi, P., Lo, K., Yu, M.C. and Jones, P.A. (1992) *Cancer Res.* **52**: 4787–4790.
68. Ooi, E.E., Ren, E.C. and Chan, S.H. (1997) *Int. J. Cancer,* **74**:, 229–232.
69. Bouvier, G., Poirier, S., Shao, Y.M., Malaveille, C., Ohshima, H., Polack, A., Bornkamm, G.W., Zeng, Y., de Thé, G. and Bartsch, H. (1991) in: *Relevance to Human Cancer of N-Nitroso Compounds, Tobacco Smoke and Mycotoxins.* (eds I.K. O'Neill, J. Chen and H. Bartsch). IARC, Lyon, pp. 204–209.
70. Yu, M.C. (1991) in *Relevance to Human Cancer of N-Nitroso Compounds, Tobacco Smoke and Mycotoxins.* (eds I.K. O'Neill, J. Chen and H. Bartsch). IARC, Lyon, pp. 39–47.
71. Zeng, Y. (1985) *Adv. Cancer Res.* **44**: 121–138.
72. Henle, W. (1971). *Proceedings of International Symposium. Princess Takamatsu Cancer Research Fund. Recent Advances in Tumour Virology Immunology.* (eds W. Nakahara, K. Nishioka, T. Hirayama and Y. Ito). University Park Press, Baltimore, pp. 361–367.

## Further reading

Frappier, L. and Bochkarev, A. (1997) EBNA1 structure. *Epstein–Barr Virus Report* **4**: 87–90.

**Fruehling, S., Caldwell, R. and Longnecker, R.** (1997) LMP2 function in EBV latency. *Epstein–Barr Virus Report* **4:** 151–159.

**Kieff, E.** (1996) Epstein–Barr virus and its replication. in *Virology*, 3rd Edn. (eds B.N. Fields, D.M. Knipe and P.M. Howley). Lippincott–Raven Press, New York, pp. 2343–2396.

**Rickinson, A.B. and Kieff, E.** (1996) in *Virology*, 3rd Edn. (eds. B.N. Fields, D.M. Knipe and P.M. Howley). Lippincott–Raven Press, New York, pp. 2397–2446.

**Robertson, E.S.** (1997) The Epstein–Barr Virus EBNA3 protein family as regulators of transcription. *Epstein–Barr Virus Report* **4:** 143–150.

Chapter 5

# Kaposi's sarcoma and human herpesvirus-8

## Denise Whitby, Nicola A. Smith and Simon J. Talbot

## 5.1 Kaposi's sarcoma

Kaposi's sarcoma (KS) was originally described by the Austro-Hungarian dermatologist Moritz Kaposi in 1872 [1]. The tumour usually appears as brownish-purple skin lesions, often on the extremities, but may in more aggressive forms of the disease progress to involve organs such as the lungs, lymph nodes and gastro-intestinal tract. The lesions contain many types of cell but are characterized histologically by the presence of elongated 'spindle' cells and irregular slit-like vascular spaces.

The origin of the spindle cells is disputed, immunohistochemistry of KS lesions has been used by many groups to demonstrate the expression of various cell markers on spindle cells. Several studies have demonstrated the expression of markers specific for lymphatic or vascular endothelial cells [2,3]. Other studies have shown expression of markers for monocytes/macrophages [4], dermal dendrocytes [5] and smooth muscle cells [6,7]. Because of the conflicting data it has been suggested that spindle cells in KS lesions may be derived from more than one cell type [8] or from a mesenchymal progenitor cell [9].

There is also controversy as to whether KS is a true malignant neoplasm as it has features of both a hyperplasia and a neoplasm (*Table 5.1*).

Four forms of KS have been described, all of which are histologically identical but are distinguished by epidemiological factors and disease severity.

### 5.1.1 Classic KS

Classic KS (*Figure 5.1*) is characterized by benign, indolent tumours often limited to the extremities. It is rare in the USA and northern Europe and occurs

*Viruses and Human Cancer*, edited by J.R. Arrand and D.R. Harper
© 1998 BIOS Scientific Publishers Ltd, Oxford

**Table 5.1.** Features of KS characteristic of a neoplasm or a reactive hyperplasia

| Features of neoplasia | Present in KS? | Features of hyperplasia | Present in KS? |
|---|---|---|---|
| Monoclonality | YES ? [10] | Polyclonality | YES |
| Transformed cell type | NO – most cell lines are not transformed | Non-transformed cells | YES – most cell lines are not transformed |
| | YES – two recent ones are | | NO – two recent ones are |
| Causes human tumours when injected into nude mice | NO – most cause tumour of mouse origin | Cause reactive tumours of mouse origin | YES |
| Metastatic | Multicentric rather than metastatic | Not metastatic | YES |

mostly in elderly men of Mediterranean, Middle Eastern or Jewish descent [11].

### 5.1.2 African, or endemic, KS

African, or endemic, KS is common in parts of sub-Saharan Africa. In adults it occurs more often in men, but unlike classic KS it is also seen in children of both sexes. It is generally a more aggressive form of KS, particularly in young children where lymph node involvement is common and the disease is rapidly fatal [12,13].

### 5.1.3 Iatrogenic KS

Iatrogenic KS occurs in individuals who are immunosuppressed because of organ transplantation [14].

### 5.1.4 AIDS-related KS

AIDS-related KS (*Figure 5.2*) is the best known form of KS. It is often very aggressive with widely disseminated cutaneous lesions, visceral involvement and associated mortality. Indeed it was the appearance of KS in young homosexual and bisexual men in the USA which was one of the first signs of the acquired immune deficiency syndrome (AIDS) epidemic [15].

Strong epidemiological evidence has accumulated over the last decade suggesting that KS is caused by a sexually transmitted infectious agent: KS is 300 times more common in AIDS patients than in other immunosuppressed groups and 20 000 times more common than in the general population. Importantly, KS is 10 times more common in homosexual or bisexual men with AIDS than in other groups of human immune deficiency virus (HIV)-infected individuals (*Figure 5.3*), who have become infected by non-sexual routes, such as indi-

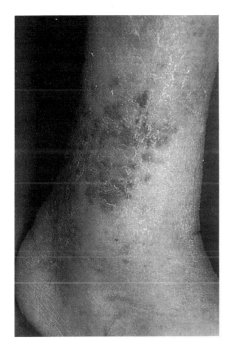 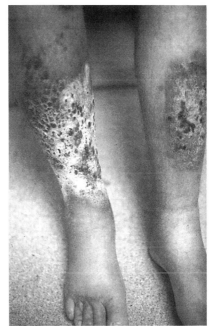

**Figure 5.1**. Typical lesion of classic Kaposi's sarcoma.

viduals with haemophilia, intravenous drug users or blood transfusion recipients [16]. KS also occurs in young gay men who are not HIV-infected [17]. In Africa, AIDS-related KS (AIDS-KS) is seen in those who acquire HIV by heterosexual contact [18].

Despite strong evidence for the association of an infectious agent with KS, numerous studies have failed to show an association with cytomegalovirus [19], human papillomavirus [20], retrovirus-like particles [21], human herpesvirus-6 [22,23], *Mycoplasma penetrans* [24] or HIV [25–27].

## 5.2 Discovery of human herpesvirus-8

Using a technique based on the polymerase chain reaction (PCR) called representational difference analysis [28], Chang *et al.* discovered a new human herpesvirus in tumour tissue from AIDS-KS [29]. It was initially given the descriptive name Kaposi's sarcoma associated herpesvirus (KSHV), but is also known as human herpesvirus-8 (HHV-8), and this term will be used throughout the chapter. Viral sequences have now been detected, using PCR, in over 95% of all KS lesions [30–33]. The entire genome (See Section 5.6) of the new virus has been cloned and sequenced and shown to be a gamma-2-herpesvirus with similarity to the human gammaherpesvirus Epstein–Barr virus (EBV) (*Figure 5.4*) [34–36].

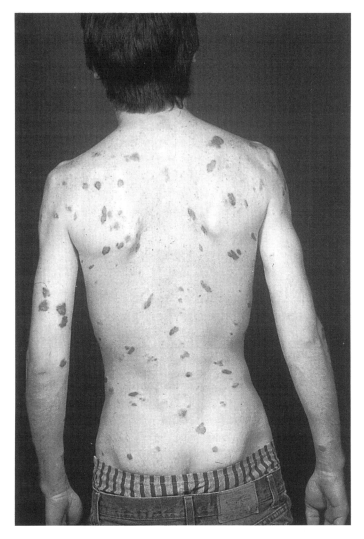

**Figure 5.2**. Typical lesions of AIDS–related Kaposi's sarcoma.

## 5.3 The prevalence of HHV-8 DNA

It has been suggested that HHV-8 may be ubiquitous in the general population, as is the case for the other human herpesviruses, and that it preferentially replicates in KS tissue without being the cause of the tumour. For this reason the prevalence of the virus in populations both affected and unaffected by KS is of crucial importance in establishing whether or not it causes KS.

Initial HHV-8 prevalence studies were based on the detection of viral DNA by PCR in biopsies of tumours and other tissues (*Table 5.2*). Further studies looked for HHV-8 DNA in the peripheral blood where the virus is present in B lymphocytes (*Table 5.3*). These studies have confirmed that HHV-8 infection parallels the occurrence of KS and that detection of HHV-8 in asymptomatic

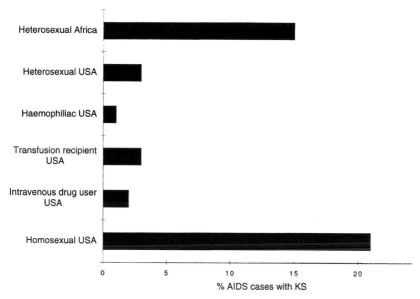

**Figure 5.3**. Prevalence of AIDS cases with Kaposi's sarcoma in different groups of HIV-infected patients.

HIV-positive individuals strongly predicts subsequent progression of those patients to development of KS [56]. These data are highly suggestive of a causal role for HHV-8 in KS. HHV-8 is also detected in some HIV-negative,

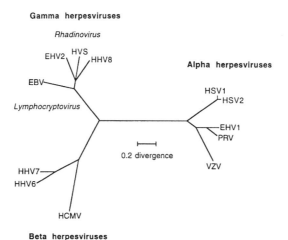

**Figure 5.4**. Phylogenetic tree showing relation of HHV-8 to other herpesviruses. Abbreviations: HSV, herpes simplex virus; EHV, equine herpesvirus; PRV, pseudorabies virus; VZV, varicella zoster virus; HCMV, human cytomegalovirus; HVS, *Herpesvirus saimiri*. The branch lengths are proportional to the divergence (mean number of substitution events per site) between the nodes bounding each branch. Redrawn from Moore et al., 1996, Journal of Virology, Volume 30, with permission from The American Society for Microbiology.

**Table 5.2.** PCR Detection of HHV-8 DNA in biopsies

| Type of KS lesion | Positive (n) | Tested (n) | Positive (%) |
|---|---|---|---|
| AIDS-KS | 252 | 259 | 97 |
| Classic KS | 160 | 175 | 91 |
| Iatrogenic KS | 13 | 13 | 100 |
| African endemic | 71 | 80 | 89 |
| HIV-negative gay men with KS | 8 | 9 | 89 |
| Control tissues | 14 | 743 | 1.8 |

Data from [29,31,33,37–55]

healthy people where its potential to cause disease is unknown but likely to be small.

HHV-8 has been detected, infrequently, in saliva of AIDS-KS patients [56,61] and also in the bronchoalveolar lavage fluid from over 80% of patients with pulmonary KS [62]. There have been no reports of detection of HHV-8 in saliva of classic KS patients or symptom-free individuals infected with HHV-8; thus the role of saliva in the transmission of HHV-8 remains unclear. HHV-8 has not been detected in the faeces of AIDS-KS patients [56] (*Table 5.4*).

Conflicting data have emerged as to the prevalence of HHV-8 in semen (*Table 5.5*). Taken together these reports suggest that sexual transmission of HHV-8 via semen is likely to occur but that HHV-8 is not prevalent outside the known KS risk groups.

There have been fewer studies examining the prevalence of HHV-8 in the female genital tract (*Table 5.5*). Two small studies reported that HHV-8 was not detected in small numbers of cervical or vulval cancer specimens in the US [67] and Italy [60]. We have completed a larger study of cervical smears from HIV-positive and -negative women from the UK, and found that HHV-8 could be detected in a proportion of women of African origin but not in others. Such detection has important implications for both sexual and vertical transmission of HHV-8.

**Table 5.3.** PCR detection of HHV-8 in peripheral blood mononuclear cells

| Type of patient | Positive (n) | Tested (n) | Positive (%) |
|---|---|---|---|
| AIDS-KS | 132 | 290 | 46 |
| Classic KS | 33 | 58 | 57 |
| African endemic KS | 33 | 38 | 87 |
| Iatrogenic KS | 0 | 2 | 0 |
| HIV-negative men with KS | 1 | 6 | 17 |
| HIV-positive without KS | 30 | 386 | 8 |
| HIV-negative without K | 0 | 368 | 0 |
| HIV-negative without KS (Italy) | 5 | 56 | 9 |

Data from [32,40–41, 55–60].

**Table 5.4.** HHV-8 DNA detection in body fluids

| Type of body fluid | Positive (n) | Tested (n) | Positive (%) |
|---|---|---|---|
| Saliva | | | |
|    AIDS-KS | 19 | 51 | 37 |
|    HIV-positive without KS | 29 | 120 | 24 |
|    HIV- negative without KS | 0 | 39 | 0 |
| Faeces | | | |
|    AIDS-KS | 0 | 18 | 0 |
| Broncho-alveolar lavage | | | |
|    AIDS-KS | 19 | 51 | 37 |

Data from [56, 62–65].

## 5.4 The prevalence of HHV-8 antibodies

First generation serological assays have been developed which detect antibodies to HHV-8 antigens expressed when the virus is actively dividing (lytic antigens) or when the virus is lying dormant (latent nuclear antigens such as LNA1; formally analogous to the EBV-encoded EBNAs). Seroprevalence of antibodies to HHV-8 is significantly higher in groups at risk for KS, such as HIV-infected gay men and also in areas such as sub-Saharan Africa and the Mediterranean where the rate of KS is relatively high [71–73]. Serological studies have also indicated that HHV-8 is sexually transmitted, since antibodies are more frequently detected in sexually transmitted diseases clinic attendees [73,74]. The prevalence of HHV-8 antibodies in the general population is controversial and studies have reported rates varying from 0 to 20% depending whether the test is for lytic or latent antibodies. This discrepancy may be due to a low sensitivity of the latent assay or a low specificity of the lytic assay. Whether the background prevalence of HHV-8 is < 1% or 20%, it is clearly much lower than in those with KS or at risk for KS, and therefore the seroepi-

**Table 5.5.** HHV-8 DNA detection in genital tract samples

| Sample type | Positive (n) | Tested (n) | Positive (%) |
|---|---|---|---|
| Semen | | | |
|    AIDS-KS | 19 | 87 | 22 |
|    Classic KS | 0 | 4 | 0 |
|    HIV-positive without KS | 7 | 78 | 9 |
|    Healthy donors | 0 | 135 | 0 |
|    Healthy donors (Italy) | 36 | 98 | 37 |
| Prostate biopsy | 9 | 85 | 11 |
| Female genital tract biopsy | 3 | 96 | 3 |
| Cervical scrape | 5 | 136 | 3.6 |

Data from [40,51,54–55,60,66–70.

**Table 5.6.** detection of antibodies to HHV-8 latent and lytic antigens

| Sera | Latent antigen assays (IFA) | | | Lytic antigen assays (IFA, WB, ORF 65 ELISA) | | |
|---|---|---|---|---|---|---|
| | Positive (n) | Tested (n) | Positive (%) | Positive (n) | Tested (n) | Positive (%) |
| AIDS KS | 228 | 312 | 73 | 156 | 244 | 64 |
| Classic KS | 29 | 30 | 97 | 17 | 18 | 94 |
| African KS | 28 | 28 | 100 | 42 | 45 | 93 |
| HIV-positive gay men without KS | 38 | 144 | 26 | 106 | 218 | 49 |
| STD clinic attendees | 40 | 357 | 11 | – | – | – |
| Controls USA/UK | 6 | 413 | 1.5 | 122 | 1207 | 10 |
| Africa | 55 | 286 | 19 | 184 | 290 | 63 |
| Greece/Italy | 7 | 133 | 5 | 3 | 26 | 12 |

Data from [72–76].
Abbreviations: IFA, immunofluorescence assay; WB, Western blot; ORF 65, open reading frame 65; ELISA, enzyme linked immunosorbent assay.

demiology of HHV-8 reported so far supports a causal role for HHV-8 in KS (*Table 5.6*).

## 5.5 HHV-8 and other diseases

HHV-8 is considered to be an aetiological agent of a rare form of AIDS-associated B-cell lymphoma, primary effusion lymphoma, also known as body-cavity-based-lymphoma, which is associated with KS [77–79]. HHV-8 has also been reported by several groups to be present in Multicentric Castleman's Disease, a lymphoproliferative disorder also frequently associated with KS [33,52,80]. Recently, HHV-8-specific DNA has been shown to be present in the bone marrow dendritic cells of multiple myeloma patients but is absent from malignant plasma cells or the dendritic cells from healthy individuals or patients with other malignancies [81]. It has been postulated that HHV-8 may be able to perpetuate the growth of the malignant plasma cells by secretion of viral interleukin-6 (vIL-6, see Section 5.9) from infected bone marrow dendritic cells, although these results have yet to be confirmed.

## 5.6 The HHV-8 genome

HHV-8 is an enveloped, double-stranded DNA virus with a genome of approximately 170 000 base pairs and belongs to the rhadinovirus subgroup of gammaherpesviruses. The complete nucleotide sequence of HHV-8 DNA has recently been determined and shown to contain 81 open reading frames (ORFs) of which 66 have sequence similarity to the genes of the oncogenic gammaherpesvirus (EBV) [36,82–83].

As with other rhadinoviruses, HHV-8 has numerous ORFs with striking similarity to known cellular genes (*Figure 5.5*). These have probably been cap-

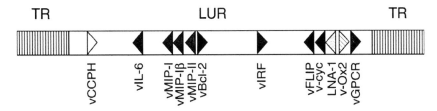

**Figure 5.5**. General organization of the HHV-8 genome showing the location of several genes of interest. The genome consists of a long unique (coding) region (LUR) flanked by terminal repeats (TR). The positions and orientations of genes referred to in the text are indicated by triangles. Genes involved in cell growth or apoptosis, v-*cyc* (D-type cyclin homologue), FLIP (FLICE inhibitory protein) and *bcl-2* are shown in black; genes related to cytokines or chemokines, vIL-6 (viral interleukin-6), vMIP-I (viral macrophage inflammatory protein), vMIP-II, vMIP-Iβ, or involved in signal transduction pathways, GPCR (G-protein-coupled receptor), IRF (interferon regulatory factor) are indicated in dark grey. CCPH (complement controlled protein homologue) is a modulator of the immune system whilst the Ox-2 homologue and LNA-1 (latent nuclear antigen) have no known functions as yet.

tured from the host cell during viral evolution and include genes encoding proteins that regulate the cell cycle or that interfere with the immune system. Such gene products could play a role in cellular transformation and tumour induction (*Table 5.7*).

## 5.7 HHV-8 genes involved in cellular proliferation

Host cell responses to viral infection include shutting down the cell cycle, induction of apoptosis [84–88] and enhancement of immune responses through up-regulation of major histocompatibility complex (MHC) antigens [89–90]. Many viruses have evolved specific proteins which can defeat these host defences [91–94].

The retinoblastoma protein (pRB) is a cellular protein that has a role in the regulation of normal cell division (see Section 3.5.1). It blocks the cell division cycle at the G1 phase and prevents progression through mitosis. The HHV-8 encoded cyclin gene (v-cyc; Orf 72) promotes phosphorylation and inactivation of pRB (primarily through activation of cdk 6). Hence the G1 cell cycle checkpoint is ineffective leading to unregulated cell division [95–97].

HHV-8 encodes a G-protein-coupled receptor (vGPCR; orf 75) that is homologous to the human interleukin (IL)-8 receptor [98–100]. It binds IL-8 with high affinity, and activates the same signal transduction cascade. However, the HHV-8 GPCR is constitutively active (i.e. it does not require activation by an agonist). There are two potential mechanisms whereby vGPCR could act in the development of HHV-8-associated diseases: directly with constitutive signalling of vGPCR leading to altered growth and neoplastic transformation, and/or indirectly, whereby signalling by vGPCR induces the expression of other genes which are involved in the pathogenesis of KS [98].

**Table 5.7.** HHV-8 genes implicated in tumorigenesis

| Host cell homologue | HHV-8 encoded protein | Possible function |
|---|---|---|
| D-type cyclin | v-Cyc | Inactivation of pRB Promotes G1 to S phase transition |
| IL-8 GPCR | v-GPCR | Cellular growth signal |
| Interferon regulatory factor | v-IRF | Inhibits p21 and MHC class I expression |
| CC chemokines | v-MIP-I, v-MIP-II v-MIP-1β | Chemoattraction, angiogenesis |
| IL-6 | v-IL-6 | Growth factor for KS cells |
| Bcl-2 family protein | v-Bcl-2 | Inhibition of apoptosis |
| FLICE inhibitory protein | v-FLIP | Inhibition of CD95L and TNF-induced apoptosis |
| N-CAM family protein | v-Ox-2 | Cellular adhesion molecule |
| CD21/CR2 complement binding protein | Orf 4 | Escape from host immune response |

Encoded on a bicistronic messenger RNA (mRNA) together with the vGPCR is a putative transmembrane protein of the N-CAM family (v-Ox2). This membrane protein is possibly involved in cell signalling and/or cell adhesion. Cell adhesion molecules such as integrins are thought to play a role in the pathogenesis of AIDS-KS, in particular through interaction with HIV Tat protein and basic fibroblast growth factor. v-Ox2 is not shared by the other gammaherpesviruses such as herpes simplex virus or EBV.

Interferon (IFN) inhibits cellular proliferation [101–103], induces apoptosis [104–105], and up-regulates MHC antigens which activate the immune response against the infected cells [106–109]. HHV-8 encodes an interferon regulatory protein homologue (vIRF; Orf K9) which can inhibit interferon-β signal transduction [76]. Inhibition of the function of cellular IFN may contribute to viral escape from immune surveillance and apoptosis.

Another ORF, Orf4, is a complement control protein homologue possibly involved in the protection of HHV-8 infected cells against killing by complement.

## 5.8 Apoptosis

The induction of apoptosis is a typical response of the host cell to virus infection. Deregulation of the host cell-cycle machinery (discussed above) by virally encoded proteins, leads to the up-regulation of the tumour suppressor protein p53. This protein activates genes encoding apoptosis-mediating proteins such as Bax and Bik [110,111]. The p53 protein also up-regulates expression of death receptors such as CD95 (Fas, Apo-1) together with its ligand CD95L (FasL) which signal a cell to apoptose [112]. HHV-8 encodes a gene (v-*bcl*-2) which can bind to, and inactivate, Bax and prevent it from inducing apoptosis. This viral protein is similar to cellular *Bcl-2* [113,114].

HHV-8 also encodes a homologue of a recently identified family of apoptosis inhibitors known as FLIPs (FLICE inhibitory proteins). These proteins interfere with apoptosis signalled through cellular death receptors. Cells expressing vFLIP are protected against apoptosis induced by signals such as CD95 or by tumour necrosis factor receptor 1 [112,115]. Protection of virus infected cells from death receptor-induced apoptosis probably leads to higher virus production and contributes to the persistence and oncogenicity of FLIP-encoding viruses.

## 5.9 Chemokines and cytokines

Human IL-6 (hIL-6) has long been suspected to be involved in the pathogenesis of KS. The expression of hIL-6 is elevated in KS lesions and cultured KS cells have been reported to respond to recombinant hIL-6 with increased growth [116–117]. HHV-8 encodes a homologue of hIL-6 [viral IL-6 (vIL-6)] [118,119].

hIL-6 has also been shown to be a growth factor for three other HHV-8-associated diseases, primary effusion lymphomas, Multicentric Castleman's Disease, and multiple myeloma [81].

Two virus proteins similar to two human macrophage inflammatory protein (MIP-1β) chemokines, and a third protein similar to both MIP-1β and macrophage chemoattractant protein chemokines have been identified in the HHV-8 genome (Orfs K4, K6 and K4.1) [83,118]. These may act as chemoattractants and angiogenesis promoters.

## 5.10 *In vitro* culture of HHV-8

Although HHV-8 is present in all KS lesions, cell cultures and cell lines derived from KS lesions lose detectable HHV-8 after a few passages. The reasons for this are unclear at present. It is possible that the HHV-8 infected spindle cells do not grow in culture, or that the culture systems employed result in HHV-8 being lost from cultured cells. By contrast several cell lines have been established from primary effusion lymphoma cells (see Section 5.5), which have been shown to be latently infected with a high number of HHV-8 genome copies per cell [78,120]. Lytic replication of HHV-8 can be induced in these cell lines using phorbol esters.

Isolation and propagation of HHV-8 in the human embryonal kidney cell line 293 has also been described [121].

## 5.11 In conclusion

Seroepidemiology and PCR studies strongly suggest that HHV-8 is the cause of KS and primary effusion lymphoma, and is also associated with

Multicentric Castleman's Disease. Although HHV-8 has not yet been shown to be a transforming virus *in vitro*, the virus encodes several proteins capable of the deregulation of cell cycle control (v-Cyc, vGPCR, vIRF), inhibition of apoptosis (vBcl-2, vFLIP) and control of growth differentiation (vIL-6, vMIP-I, vMIP-II, vMIP-Iβ), which could contribute to tumour formation.

## References

1. **Kaposi, M.** (1872) Arch. *Dermatol Syphillis* **4**: 265–273.
2. **Beckstead, J.H., Wood, G.S. and Fletcher, V.** (1985) *Am. J. Pathol.* **119**: 294–300.
3. **Rutgers, J.L., Wieczorek, R., Bonetti, F., Kaplan, K.L., Posnett, D.N., Friedman-Kien, A.E. and Knowles, D.M.** (1986) *Am. J. Pathol.* **122**: 493–499.
4. **Uccini, S., Ruco, L.P., Monardo, F., Stoppacciaro, A., Dejana, E., La Parola, I.L., Cerimele, D. and Baroni, C.D.** (1994) *J. Pathol.* **173**: 23–31.
5. **Nickoloff, B. J. and Griffiths, C.E.** (1989) *Science.* **243**: 1736–1737.
6. **Thompson, E.W., Nakamura, S., Shima, T.B., Melchiori, A., Martin, G.R., Salahuddin, S.Z., Gallo, R.C. and Albini, A.** (1991) *Cancer Res.* **51**: 2670–2676.
7. **Weich, H.A., Salahuddin, S.Z., Gill, P., Nakamura, S., Gallo, R.C. and Folkmann, J.** (1991) *Am. J. Pathol.* **139**: 1251–1258.
8. **Roth, W.K.** (1991) *J. Cancer Res. Clin. Oncol.* **117**: 186–191.
9. **Weiss, R.A.** (1996) *Nature Med.* **2**: 277–278.
10. **Rabkin, C.S., Janz, S., Lash, A., Coleman, A.E., Musaba, E., Liotta, L., Biggar, R.J. and Zhuang, Z.** (1997) *New Engl. J. Med.* **336**: 988–993.
11. **Wahman, A., Melnick, S.L., Rhame, F.S. and Potter, J.D.** (1991) *Epidemiol. Rev.* **13**: 178–199.
12. **Taylor, J.F., Smith, P.G., Bull, D. and Pike, M.C.** (1972) *Br. J. Cancer* **26**: 483–497.
13. **Ziegler, J.L. and Katongole Mbidde, E.** (1996) *Int. J. Cancer* **65**: 200–203.
14. **Farge, D., Herve, R., Mikol, J.** *et al.* (1994) *Leukaemia* **8**: 318–321.
15. **Beral, V., Peterman, T.A., Berkelman, R.L. and Jaffe, H.W.** (1990) *Lancet* **335**: 123–128.
16. **Beral, V.** (1991) in *Cancer, HIV and AIDS.* (eds V. Beral, H.W. Jaffe and R.A. Weiss). Cold Spring Harbor Laboratory Press, New York, pp. 5–22.
17. **Friedman Kien, A.E., Saltzman, B.R., Cao, Y.Z., Nestor, M.S., Mirabile, M., Li, J.J. and Peterman, T.A.** (1990) *Lancet* **335**: 168–169.
18. **Beral, V., Jaffe, H.W. and Weiss, R.A.** (1990) *Cancer Surveys 1990: Cancer, HIV and AIDS* . Cold Spring Harbor Laboratory Press, New York, pp. 1–112.
19. **Giraldo, G., Beth, E. and Kyalwazi, S.K.** (1984) *IARC Scientific Publications* **63**: 583–606.
20. **Huang, Y.Q., Li, J.J., Rush, M.G., Poiesz, B.J., Nicolaides, A., Jacobson, M., Zhang, W.G., Coutavas, E., Abbott, M.A. and Friedman Kien, A.E.** (1992) *Lancet* **339**: 515–518.
21. **Rappersberger, K., Tschachler, E., Zonzits, E.** *et al.* (1990) *J. Inv. Dermatol.* **95**: 371–381.
22. **Kempf, W. and Adams, V.** (1996) *Biochem. Mol. Med.* **58**: 1–12.
23. **Kempf, W., Adams, V., Pfaltz, M., Briner, J., Schmid, M., Moos, R. and Hassam, S.** (1995) *Hum. Pathol.* **26**: 914–919.

24. **Wang, R.Y.H., Shih, J.W.K., Weiss, S.H.,** *et al.* (1993) *Clin. Inf. Dis.* **17:** 724–729.
25. **Barillari, G., Buonaguro, L., Fiorelli, V., Hoffman, J., Michaels, F., Gallo, R.C. and Ensoli, B.** (1992) *J. Immunol.* **149:** 3727–3734.
26. **Ensoli, B., Barillari, G., Salahuddin, S.Z., Gallo, R.C., and Wong, S.F.** (1990) *Nature* **345:** 84–86.
27. **Ensoli, B., Gendelman, R., Markham, P., Fiorelli, V., Colombini, S., Raffeld, M., Cafaro, A., Chang, H.K., Brady, J.N. and Gallo, R.C. (1994).** *Nature* **371:** 674–680.
28. **Lisitsyn, N., Lisitsyn, N. and Wigler, M.** (1993) *Science* **259:** 946-951.
29. **Chang, Y., Cesarman, E., Pessin, M.S., Lee, F., Culpepper, J., Knowles, D.M., and Moore, P.S. (1994).** *Science* **266:** 1865–1869.
30. **Boshoff, C., Whitby, D., Hatziioannou, T., Fisher, C., van der Walt, J., Hatzakis, A., Weiss, R. and Schulz, T.** (1995) *Lancet* **345:** 1043–1044.
31. **Chang, Y., Ziegler, J., Wabinga, H.** *et al.* (1996) *Arch. Int. Med.* **156:** 202–204.
32. **Collandre, H., Ferris, S., Grau, O., Montagnier, L. and Blanchard, A.** (1995) *Lancet* **345:** 1043.
33. **Dupin, N., Gorin, I., Deleuze, J., Agut, H., Huraux, J.M. and Escande, J.P.** (1995) *N. Engl. J. Med.* **333:** 798–799.
34. **Moore, P.S., Gao, S.J., Dominguez, G., Cesarman, E., Lungu, O., Knowles, D.M., Garber, R., Pellett, P.E., McGeoch, D.J. and Chang, Y.** (1996) *J. Virol.* **70:** 549–558.
35. **Neipel, F., Albrecht, J.C., Ensser, A., Huang, Y.Q., Li, J.J., Friedman Kien, A. E. and Fleckenstein, B.** (1997) Primary structure of the Kaposi's sarcoma associated human herpesvirus 8. Genbank accession no. U93872.
36. **Russo, J.J., Bohenzky, R.A., Chien, M.C., Chen, J., Yan, M., Maddalena, D., Parry, J.P., Peruzzi, D., Edelman, I.S., Chang, Y. and Moore, P.S.** (1996) *Proc. Natl Acad. Sci. USA* **93:** 14862–14867.
37. **Su, J., Hsu, Y.S., Chang, Y.C. and Wang, I.W.** (1995) *Lancet* **345:** 722–723.
38. **Huang, Y.Q., Li, J.J., Kaplan, M.H., Poiesz, B., Katabira, E., Zhang, W.C., Feiner, D. and Friedman-Kien, A.E.** (1995) *Lancet* **345:** 759–761.
39. **Boshoff, C., Schulz, T.F., Kennedy, M.M., Graham, A.K., Fisher, C., Thomas, A., McGee Od, J., Weiss, R.A. and Oleary, J.J.** (1995) *Nature Med.* **1:** 1274–1278.
40. **Ambroziak, J.A., Blackbourn, D.J., Herndier, B.G., Glogau, R.G., Gullett, J.H., McDonald, A.R., Lennette, E.T. and Levy, J.A.** (1995) *Science* **268:** 582–583.
41. **Moore, P.S., Kingsley, L.A., Holmberg, S.D., Spira, T., Gupta, P., Hoover, D.R., Parry, J.P., Conley, L.J., Jaffe, H.W. and Chang, Y.** (1996) *AIDS* **10:** 175–180.
42. **Lebbe, C., de Cremoux, P., Rybojad, M, Costa da Cunha, C., Morel, P. and Calvo, F.** (1995) *Lancet* **345:** 1180.
43. **Schalling, M., Ekman, M., Kaaya, E.E., Linde, A. and Biberfeld, P.** (1995) *Nature Med.* **1:** 705–706.
44. **Chuck, S., Grant, R.M., Katongole-Mbidde, E., Conant, M. and Ganem, D.** (1996) *J. Infect. Dis.* **173:** 248–251.
45. **O'Neill, E., Henson, T.H., Ghorbani, A.J., Land, M.A., Webber, B.L. and Garcia, J.V.** (1996) *J. Clin. Pathol.* **49:** 306–308.
46. **Buonaguro, F.M., Tornesello, M.L., Beth-Giraldo, E., Hatzakis, A., Mueller, N., Downing, R., Biryamwaho, B., Sempala, S.D. and Giraldo, G.** (1996) *Int. J. Cancer* **65:** 25–28.

47. Cathomas, G., McGandy, C.E., Terracciano, L.M., Itin, P.H., de Rosa, G. and Gudat, F. (1996) *J. Clin. Pathol.* **49**: 631–633.

48. Gaidano, G., Pastore, C., Gloghini, A. et al. (1996) *AIDS* **10**: 941–949.

49. Jin Y.T., Tsai, S.T., Yan, J.J., Hsiao, J.H., Lee, Y.Y. and Su, I.J. (1996) *Am. J. Clin. Path.* **105**: 360–363.

50. Dictor, M., Rambech, E., Way, D., Witte, M. and Bendsoe, N. (1996) *Am. J. Pathol.* **148**: 2009–2016.

51. Marchioli, C.C., Love, J.L., Abbott, L.Z., Huang, Y.Q., Remick, S.C., Surtento-Reodica, N., Hutchison, R.E., Mildvan, D., Friedman-Kien, A.E. and Poiesz, B.J. (1996) *J. Clin. Microbiol.* **34**: 2635–2638.

52. Luppi, M., Barozzi, P., Maiorana, A., Artusi, T., Trovato, R., Marasca, R., Savarino, M., Ceccherini Nelli, L. and Torelli, G. (1996) *Blood* **87**: 3903–3909.

53. McDonagh, D.P., Liu, J., Gaffey, M.J., Layfield, L.J., Azumi, N. and Traweek, T. S. (1996) *Am. J. Pathol.* **149**: 1363–1368.

54. Corbellino, M., Bestetti, G., Poirel, L., Aubin, J. T., Brambilla, L., Pizzuto, M., Capra, M., Berti, E., Galli, M. and Parravicini, C. (1996) *J. Infect. Dis.* **174**: 668–670.

55. Lebbe, C., Agbalika, F., de Cremoux, P., Deplanche, M., Rybojad, M., Masgrau, E., Morel, P. and Calvo, F. (1997) *Arch. Dermatol.* **133**: 25–30.

56. Whitby, D., Howard, M.R., Tenant Flowers, M. *et al.* (1995) *Lancet* **346**: 799–802.

57. Bigoni, B., Dolcetti, R., de Lellis, L., Carbone, A., Boiocchi, M., Cassai, E. and Di Luca, D. (1996) *J. Infect. Dis.* **173**: 542–549.

58. Humphrey, R.W., O'Brien, T.R., Newcomb, F.M., Nishihara, H., Wyvill, K.M., Ramos, G.A., Saville, M.W., Goedert, J.J., Straus, S.E. and Yarchoan, R. (1996) *Blood* **88**: 297–301.

59. Purvis, S.F., Katongole-Mbidde, E., Johnson, J.L., Leonard, D.G., Bybazaire, N., Luckey, C., Schick, H.E., Wallis, R., Elmets, C.A. and Giam, C.Z. (1997) *J. Infect. Dis.* **175**: 947–950.

60. Viviano, E., Vitale, F., Ajello, F., Perna, A.M., Villafrate, M.R., Bonura, F., Arico, M., Mazzola, G. and Romano, N. (1997) *AIDS* **11**: 607–612.

61. Luppi, M., Barozzi, P., Maiorana, A., Collina, G., Ferrari, M.G., Marasca, R., Morselli, M., Rossi, E., Ceccherini-Nelli, L. and Torelli, G. (1996) *Int. J. Cancer* **66**: 427–431.

62. Howard, M., Brink, N., Miller, R. and Tedder, R. (1995) *Lancet* **346**: 712.

63. Boldogh, I., Szaniszlo, P., Bresnahan, W.A., Flaitz, C.M., Nichols, M.C. and Albrecht, T. (1996) *Clin. Infect. Dis.* **23**: 406–407.

64. Koelle, D.M., Huang, M-L., Chandran, B., Vieira, J., Piepkorn, M. and Corey, L. (1997) *J. Infect. Dis.* **176**: 94–102.

65. Benfield, T.L., Dodt, K.K. and Lundgren, J.D. (1997) *Scand.J. Infect. Dis.* **29**: 13–16.

66. Monini, P., de Lellis, L., Fabris, M., Rigolin, F. and Cassai, E. (1996) *New Engl. J. Med.* **334**: 1168–1172.

67. Tasaka, T., Said, J.W. and Koeffler, H.P. (1996) *New Engl. J. Med.* **335**: 1237–1238.

68. Gupta, P., Singh, M.K., Rinaldo, C., Ding, M., Farzadegan, H., Saah, A., Hoover, D., Moore, P. and Kingsley, L. (1996) *AIDS* **10**: 1596–1598.

69. Howard, M.R., Whitby, D., Bahadur, G. *et al.* (1997) *AIDS* **11**: F15–F19.

70. Huang, Y.Q., Li, J.J. , Poiesz, B.J., Kaplan, M.H. and Friedman-Kien, A.E. (1997) *Am. J. Pathol.* **150**: 147–153.
71. Gao, S.J., Kingsley, L., Li, M. *et al.* (1996) *Nature Med.* **2**: 925–928.
72. Lennette, E.T., Blackbourn, D.J. and Levy, J.A. (1996) *Lancet* **348**: 858–861
73. Simpson, G.R., Schulz, T.F., Whitby, D. *et al.* (1996) *Lancet* **348**: 1133–1138.
74. Kedes, D. H., Operskalski, E., Busch, M., Kohn, R., Flood, J. and Ganem, D. (1996) *Nature Med.* **2**: 918–924.
75. Miller, G., Rigsby, M.O., Heston, L., Grogan, E., Sun, R., Metroka, C., Levy, J.A., Gao, S.J., Chang, Y. and Moore, P. (1996) *New Engl. J. Med.* **334**: 1292–1297.
76. Gao, S.J., Boshoff, C., Jayachandra, S., Weiss, R.A., Chang, Y. and Moore, P.S. (1997) *Oncogene* **15**: 1979–1985.
77. Ansari, M.Q., Dawson, D.B., Nador, R., Rutherford, C., Schneider, N.R., Latimer, M.J., Picker, L., Knowles, D.M. and McKenna, R.W. (1996) *Am. J. Clin. Pathol.* **105**: 221–229.
78. Cesarman, E., Moore, P.S., Rao, P.H., Inghirami, G., Knowles, D.M. and Chang, Y. (1995) *Blood* **86**: 2708–2714.
79. Chang, Y., Ziegler, J., Wabinga, H. *et al.* (1996) *Arch. Intern. Med.* **156**: 202–204.
80. Soulier, J., Grollet, L., Oksenhendler, E. *et al.* (1995) *Blood* **86**: 1276–1280.
81. Rettig, M.B., Ma, H.J., Vescio, R.A. *et al.* (1997) *Science* **276**: 1851–1854.
82. Albrecht, J. C., Nicholas, J., Biller, D. *et al.* (1992) *J. Virol.* **66**: 5047–5058.
83. Neipel, F., Albrecht, J.-C. and Fleckenstein, B. (1997) *J. Virol.* **71**: 4187–4192.
84. Dittmer, D. and Mocarski, E.S. (1997) *J. Virol.* **71**: 1629–1634.
85. Hinshaw, V.S., Olsen, C.W., Dybdahl Sissoko, N. and Evans, D. (1994) *J. Virol.* **68**: 3667–3673.
86. Shen, Y. and Shenk, T. (1996) *Proc. Nat Acad. Sci. USA* **91**: 8940–8944.
87. Shen, Y. and Shenk, T.E. (1995) *Curr. Opin. Genet. Dev.* **5**: 105–111.
88. Vaux, D.L., Haecker, G. and Strasser, A. (1994) *Cell* **76**: 777–779.
89. Biron, C.A. (1994) *Curr. Opin. Immunol.* **6**: 530–538.
90. Bot, A., Reichlin, A., Isobe, H., Bot, S., Schulman, J., Yokoyama, W.M. and Bona, C.A. (1996) *J. Virol.* **70**: 5668–5672.
91. Gooding, L.R. (1994) *Infect. Agents Dis.* **3**: 106–115.
92. Gooding, L.R. (1992) *Cell* **71**: 5–7.
93. Jagus, R. and Gray, M.M. (1994) *Biochimie* **76**: 779–791.
94. Morris, J.D., Eddleston, A.L. and Crook, T. (1995) *Lancet* **346**: 754–758.
95. Chang, Y., Moore, P.S., Talbot, S.J., Boshoff, C.H., Zarkowska, T., Godden, K., Paterson, H., Weiss, R.A. and Mittnacht, S. (1996) *Nature* **382**: 410.
96. Godden-Kent, D., Talbot, S.J., Boshoff, C., Chang, Y., Moore, P., Weiss, R.A., and Mittnacht, S. (1997) *J. Virol.* **71**: 4193–4198.
97. Li, M., Lee, H., Yoon, D.W., Albrecht, J.C., Fleckenstein, B., Neipel, F. and Jung, J.U. (1997) *J. Virol.* **71**: 1984–1991.
98. Arvanitakis, L., GerasRaaka, E., Varma, A., Gershengorn, M.C. and Cesarman, E. (1997) *Nature* **385**: 347–349.
99. Cesarman, E., Nador, R.G., Bai, F., Bohenzky, R.A., Russo, J.J., Moore, P.S., Chang, Y and Knowles, D.M. (1996) *J. Virol.* **70**: 8218–8223.
100. Guo, H.G., Browning, P., Nicholas, J. *et al.* (1997) *Virology* **228**: 371–378.
101. Kirchhoff, S., Koromilas, A.E., Schaper, F. Grashoff, M., Sonenberg, N. and Hauser, H. (1995) *Oncogene* **11**: 439–445.
102. Kirchhoff, S., Schaper, F. and Hauser, H. (1993) *Nucleic Acids Res.* **21**: 2881–2889.

103. Vaughan, P.S., Aziz, F., van Wijnen, A.J., Wu, S., Harada, H., Taniguchi, T., Soprano, K.J., Stein, J.L. and Stein, G.S. (1995) *Nature* **377**: 362–365.
104. Tamura, T., Ueda, S., Yoshida, M., Matsuzaki, M., Mohri, H. and Okubo, T. (1996) *Biochem. Biophys. Res. Comm.* **229**: 21–26.
105. Tanaka, N., Ishihara, M., Kitagawa, M., Harada, H., Kimura, T., Matsuyama, T., Lamphier, M.S., Aizawa, S., Mak, T.W. and Taniguchi, T. (1994) *Cell* **77**: 829–839.
106. Kamijo, R., Harada, H., Matsuyama, T. *et al.* (1994) *Science* **263**: 1612–1615.
107. Kimura, T., Nakayama, K., Penninger, J. *et al.* (1994) *Science* **264**: 1921–1924.
108. Martin, E., Nathan, C. and Xie, Q.W. (1994) *J. Exp. Med.* **180**: 977–984.
109. Sen, G.C. and Ransohoff, R.M. (1993) *Adv. Virus Res.* **42**: 57–102.
110. Boyd, J.M., Gallo, G.J., Elangovan, B. *et al.* (1995) *Oncogene* **11**: 1921–1928.
111. Sato, T., Hanada, M., Bodrug, S. *et al.* (1994) *Proc. Natl Acad. Sci. USA* **91**: 9238–9242.
112. Thome, M., Schneider, P., Hofmann, K. *et al.* (1997) *Nature* **386**: 517–521.
113. Cheng, E.H.Y., Nicholas, J., Bellows, D.S., Hayward, G.S., Guo, H.G., Reitz, M.S. and Hardwick, J.M. (1997) *Proc. Natl Acad. Sci. USA* **94**: 690–694.
114. Sarid, R., Sato, T., Bohenzky, R.A., Russo, J.J. and Chang, Y. (1997) *Nature Med.* **3**: 293–298.
115. Bertin, J., Armstrong, R.C., Ottilie, S., *et al.* (1997) *Proc. Natl Acad. Sci. USA* **94**: 1172–1176.
116. Miles, S.A. (1994) *Curr. Opin. Oncol.* **6**: 497–502.
117. Scala, G., Ruocco, M.R., Ambrosino, C., Mallardo, M., Giordano, V., Baldassarre, F., Dragonetti, E., Quinto, I. and Venuta, S. (1994) *J. Exp. Med.* **179**: 961–971.
118. Moore, P.S., Boshoff, C., Weiss, R.A. and Chang, Y. (1996) *Science* **274**: 1739–1744.
119. Neipel, F., Albrecht, J.C., Ensser, A., Huang, Y.Q., Li, J.J., Friedman Kien, A. E. and Fleckenstein, B. (1997) *J. Virol.* **71**: 839–842.
120. Renne, R., Zhong, W., Herndier, B., McGrath, M., Abbey, N., Kedes, D., and Ganem, D. (1996) *Nature Med.* **2**: 342–346.
121. Foreman, K.E., Friborg J., J, Kong, W.P., Woffendin, C., Polverini, P.J., Nickoloff, B.J. and Nabel, G.J. (1997) *New Engl. J. Med.* **336**: 163–171.

Chapter 6

# Human oncoretroviruses

## Graham P. Taylor and Myra McClure

## 6.1 Perspective

The *Retroviridae* are a large family of animal and human RNA viruses which replicate in infected cells via a DNA intermediate, resulting from the activity of the enzyme reverse transcriptase (RT), a virally encoded RNA-directed DNA polymerase. In humans, and in both naturally and experimentally infected animals, retroviruses can give rise to lifelong viraemia, with or without ill effects. Clinical manifestations of retroviral infection include the development of malignancies, immunosuppression and inflammatory syndromes. Despite the variety of host species infectible by retroviruses (all vertebrates, as well as some insects, fish and molluscs) and the diversity of clinical sequelae, all retroviruses share a common gross morphology, particle structure and replication cycle.

Retroviruses were traditionally classified into three subfamilies on the basis of their morphology, as defined by electron microscopy. These were: the oncoviruses (*Figure 6.1*), the lentiviruses and the foamy (spuma) viruses. The oncoviruses were a particularly mismatched group encompassing retroviruses which were oncogenic (such as murine leukaemia virus) and those that were not, such as the primate Mason–Pfizer monkey virus. Furthermore this subfamily incorporated the human leukaemia viruses [human T-lymphotropic viruses types I and II, (HTLV)I and -II] which shared more in terms of their genomic organization and disease patterns with the lentiviruses than with the oncoviruses. More recently, therefore, the International Committee on the Taxonomy of Viruses has updated retroviral classification on the basis of genomic organization and nucleotide sequences to define seven genera [1], (*Figure 6.2*), of which HTLV and like viruses (e.g. bovine leukaemia virus, BLV) constitute one genus, causing T-cell leukaemia/lymphoma and neurological disease in man and B-cell leukaemia/lymphoma in cattle and sheep. In common with other retroviruses, the HTLV virion is enveloped, surrounds two copies of single-stranded genomic RNA, targets a specific cellular receptor on the host cell and replicates via a proviral DNA intermediate.

*Viruses and Human Cancer*, edited by J.R. Arrand and D.R. Harper
© 1998 BIOS Scientific Publishers Ltd, Oxford

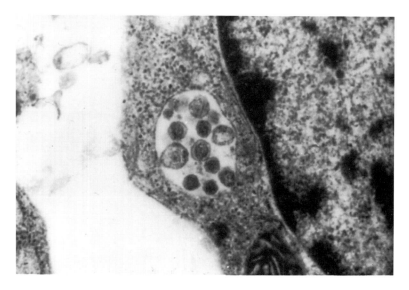

**Figure 6.1.** Electronmicrograph of HTLV-I budding from MT-2 cells. Courtesy of Dr Ian Chrystie, Department of Virology, Guys and St. Thomas's Medical School, London.

## 6.2 Historical aspects and the search for human retroviruses

It is interesting to find that the very public disputes, which have been a feature of the new discipline of human retrovirology, concerning the first isolation of the causative agent of the acquired immune deficiency syndrome (AIDS) and subsequently whether the human immunodeficiency virus type 1 (HIV-1) could cause the profound CD4+ lymphocyte depletion seen in advanced disease, only continue a trend as old as medicine itself. John Hughes Bennett in Edinburgh and Rudolph Virchow in Berlin were the first to describe the pathology of leukaemia, each conducting and reporting the first post mortems on patients with this condition within 6 weeks of each other. Their detailed reports included microscopic examination of the white cells which dominated the blood, Virchow adopting the term leukhemia whilst Bennett preferred leukocythaemia. Their dispute over priority was apparently not settled until 1858, some 13 years after their initial reports [3], with honour shared: Bennett pipping Virchow to the first report but conceding ground on the interpretation of the findings.

That leukaemia may have an infectious origin was a widely held view which gained credence when Ellerman and Bang [4] demonstrated that it could be transmitted to healthy chickens from chickens with leukaemia using cell-free extracts. This observation preceded the more renowned work of Peyton Rous [5] with chicken sarcoma in 1911 but it was not until 1951 that Gross [6] first demonstrated that mammalian leukaemia could be transmitted in mice. The first retrovirus to be described was equine infectious anaemia virus (EIAV) in 1904 [7]. However, it was not classified with this group of viruses until much later, since prior to the discovery of RT, retroviruses were called RNA tumour viruses

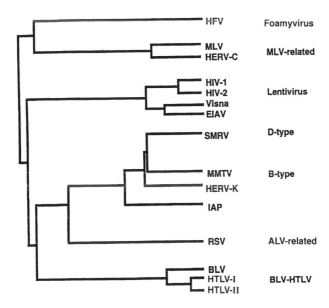

**Figure 6.2.** Seven genera of retroviruses as classified by genomic organization and nucleotide sequences. Abbreviations: HFV, human foamyvirus; MLV, murine leukaemia virus; HERV-C, human endogenous retrovirus-c; HIV, human immuno deficiency virus; EIAV, equine infectious anaemia virus; SMRV, squirrel monkey retrovirus; MMTV, mouse mammary tumour virus; HERV-K, human endogenous retrovirus-K; IAP, intracysternal A particle; RSV, Rous sarcoma virus; BLV, bovine leukaemia virus; MLV, murine leukaemia virus; ALV, avian leukaemia virus. (From [2], with permission).

and EIAV is non-oncogenic. Retroviruses were isolated from a variety of animal species over the next six decades but it was not until 1978 [8] that the first unambiguous human retrovirus was discovered. A number of investigative landmarks were critical to that achievement. The first was the identification of RT, the RNA-dependent DNA polymerase, responsible for the conversion of genomic RNA to proviral DNA. While the existence of the provirus had been theoretically implied, it was the discovery of RT by Temin [9] and Baltimore [10] which laid the cornerstone of modern retrovirology. Although not responsible for identification of this key enzyme in retroviral replication, Gallo's contribution to human retrovirology cannot be underestimated. In the face of much scepticism from the scientific community about the existence of human retroviruses, let alone retroviruses which might be associated with any human pathology, Gallo was almost alone among investigators in his unshakeable belief in their existence, their pathogenic potential and in his tenacious search for confirmatory scientific evidence. To this end he defined *in vitro* dependence of T cells on T-lymphocyte growth factor or interleukin (IL-2) [11], thus making long-term culture of those cells that support the replication of the first known human retroviruses, HTLV and HIV, possible for the first time. This, of course, was a prerequisite to their discovery. Moreover, he refined the assays of RT activity to a level of sensitivity that would allow the detection of retroviral replication *in vitro*. The stage was thus set for the discovery of HTLV and, subsequently, HIV. In 1978 his group isolated a retrovirus from the cultured cells of a patient with a cutaneous T-cell lymphoma (originally thought to be an aggressive form of mycosis fungoides, but now considered to have been the lymphomatous form of ATLL) [8]. Meanwhile a new disease, adult T-cell leukaemia (ATLL), had been described in Japan [12]. A striking characteristic of this disease was its geographical clustering with the vast majority of cases reported from southwest Japan which suggested an environmental or infectious aetiology. Once the similarity between ATLL and the cutaneous T-cell lymphoma from which HTLV had been isolated had been recognized, collaboration between the two groups revealed that the Japanese patients had antibodies to HTLV. A retrovirus, the adult T-cell leukaemia virus (ATLV) was isolated from HUT102 cells, a cell line derived in 1981 from a patient with ATLL [13]. Analysis of the RNA base sequence showed that ATLV was almost identical to HTLV [14]. In 1982 a second human retrovirus, HTLV-II, was isolated from a patient with an atypical (T cell) hairy cell leukaemia [15]. Because of these associations HTLVs are sometimes known as human T-cell leukaemia viruses.

Although HTLV-I is now recognized as the first human retrovirus to be discovered it was not always thus. A foamy virus was isolated from cultures of a nasopharyngeal carcinoma from a Kenyan patient in 1973 [16]. Foamy viruses persistently infect many mammalian species but whether they cause disease is less certain. Whilst genuine infections of humans by foamy viruses have been documented [17–18], these have usually occurred among those who handle, are bitten or scratched by non-human primates. A number of seroepidemiological studies conducted during the 1980s and early 1990s reported that antibodies to human foamy viruses were common among diverse populations [19–21]. These studies, however, lacked specificity. Recently two independent groups have carried out an extensive serological study (a combined sample size of greater than 10 000 individuals) and concluded that the apparent anti-human foamy virus (HFV) reactivity found in screening assays could not be confirmed with more specific confirmatory assays, including Western blot and polymerase chain reaction (PCR) [22–23]. Taken together with the close phylogenetic relationship with the foamy viruses isolated from chimpanzees this raises doubts as to whether a true HFV exists.

## 6.3 The human T-lymphotropic viruses

### 6.3.1 Disease associations

HTLV-I-associated diseases may be described in four categories: malignant, inflammatory, immunosuppressive, and associated with a deleted provirus.

*Malignant*. ATLL was first described as a distinct entity in Japan in 1977 [12] although the first two cases were reported in 1974 [24]. It has several distinct forms but is characterized by the presence of mature T lymphocytes which express the cell differentiation markers CD4 (helper/inducer) and CD25 (IL-2 receptor). In the leukaemic forms the presence of characteristic polylobated lymphocytes or 'flower cells' (*Figure 6.3*) aid the microscopic diagnosis, but this can be more difficult in the lymphomatous presentation. Diagnosis is usually made on microscopic and immunohistochemical analysis and by the serological confirmation of infection with HTLV-I. In doubtful cases detection of the clonal integration of HTLV-I into the expanded lymphocyte population by Southern blot or inverse PCR may be necessary to distinguish ATLL from other T-cell lymphomas in patients coincidentally infected with HTLV-I.

Patients with chronic ATLL develop the acute form within months or years. The mean survival from diagnosis of acute ATLL is 6–12 months. Immunosuppression appears more serious in ATLL than other haematological malignancies with substantial morbidity from opportunistic infections.

ATLL has been epidemiologically associated with HTLV-I infection in early life [25], either by intra-uterine transmission, infection during birth or by breast feeding. Rare cases of ATLL, have been associated with infection by blood transfusion [26]. It is however reasonable to presume that infection of the mother due to blood transfusion, during gestation or lactation with

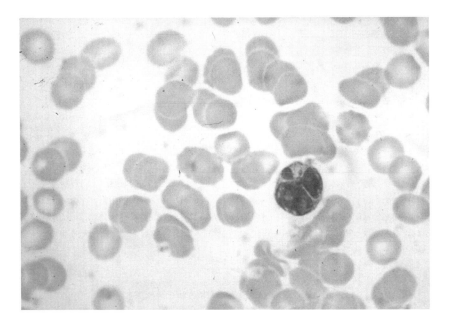

**Figure 6.3.** A polylobated lymphocyte or 'flower cell'. Courtesy of Dr Barbara Bain, Department of Haematology, Imperial College School of Medicine at St Mary's, London, UK.

subsequent mother-to-child transmission, or infection of the infant from blood transfusion would be associated with the development of ATLL, albeit many decades later. Whilst the lifetime risk of developing ATLL in all carriers is about 2%, if infection is acquired perinatally the risk is 4% [24]. Between 70 and 80% of all T-cell leukaemias that occur in the Caribbean are due to HTLV-I.

It has been suggested that in some cases of ATLL there may be synergy between HTLV and Epstein–Barr virus (EBV) (see Section 4.8.7). Whilst some reports of an increased risk of malignancy with HTLV-I infection are confounded by association with transfusion, HTLV-I infection has been linked with both an increased risk for, and an increased severity of, cervical carcinoma in Japanese [27] and Jamaican studies [28]. This association was not seen with other gynaecological malignancies and suggests synergy between human papillomavirus (Chapter 3) and HTLV-I.

Similarly, an increased frequency of hepatocellular carcinoma (HCC) has been described in patients infected with hepatitis C virus (see Section 2.7.3) and HTLV-I. In a study of chronic hepatitis due to HCV the seroprevalence of HTLV-I in those who progressed to HCC was 31% compared with 10% in those with chronic hepatitis only ($P = 0.0002$) [29]. In the Miyazaki cohort study, a prospective study in an HTLV-I endemic area which began in 1984, the relative risk for liver cancer in the HTLV-I infected group is 3.9 and 3.4 for leukaemia (non-ATLL), lymphoma, cervical carcinoma and liver cancer combined ($P = 0.03$) [30].

There are isolated reports of Kaposi's Sarcoma (KS) (associated with human herpes virus type 8, Chapter 5) occurring in patients with ATLL [31–32]. We have treated an HIV-1 and HIV-2-negative, HTLV-I-positive (serology and PCR) patient from the Gambia with 'classical' KS, (Pasvol, unpublished data). Even prior to AIDS, an increased frequency of KS had been described in patients with immunosuppression [33] (see Section 6.3.1.3, below).

**Inflammatory conditions.** These are characterized by lymphocytic infiltration of the affected tissue, and a high proviral load.

Tropical spastic paraparesis (TSP) was first associated with HTLV-I in 1985 [34] and an identical condition, HTLV-I-associated myelopathy (HAM), in Japan shortly afterwards [35]. HAM/TSP develops, on average, one decade earlier than ATLL, is more common in females and is clearly associated with transfusion-acquired infection. Up to 20% of patients with HAM/TSP in Japan and Martinique have had a blood transfusion during the 5 years prior to presentation [36] and the mean duration from infected transfusion to onset of HAM is about 3 years. Even in Europe there are several well-documented cases of HAM/TSP developing following HTLV-I infected transfusions including the case of a cardiac transplant recipient who also infected his wife [37, 38]. Other inflammatory conditions associated with HTLV-I are summarized in *Table 6.1.*

**Table 6.1.** Inflammatory disease associated with HTLV-I

| Condition | Tissue affected | Clinical presentation | Comments | References |
|---|---|---|---|---|
| Uveitis | Eye | Reduced vision | In Japan 38.8% of patients with non-specific uveitis have HTLV-I c.f. 8.4% of general population | [39–44] |
| Polymyositis | Muscle | Weakness and wasting of muscles. High serum CPK | 85% of patients with polymyositis in Caribbean and 28% in Japan have HTLV-I | [45–46] |
| Alveolitis | Lung | Cough and shortness of breath. May be asymptomatic | Most commonly described in patients with HAM/TSP | [47–48] |
| Arthropathy | Joints | Swollen large joints especially the knee | | [49–52] |
| Sjögren's syndrome | Exocrine glands | Dry eyes and mouth | Similar condition found in Tax transgenic mice | [42,53–55] |
| Infective dermatitis | Skin | Appearance of chronically infected ezcema | 14 out of 14 children in Trinidad. Treated with antibiotics longterm. ATL may develop | [56–57] |
| Autoimmune thyroiditis | Thyroid | | Three times more common than expected in Japan | [58–59] |

CPK, creatine phosphokinase

***HTLV-I and immunosuppression.*** Carriage of the helminth *Strongyloides stercoralis* is more common in HTLV-I-positive subjects [60–61] and represents a failure to clear, rather than an increased risk of, infection [62]. Hyperinfestation with *S. stercoralis* is well documented and often fails to respond to prolonged anti-parasitic therapy [63]. There is evidence of decreased suppression of EBV-infected B cells (see Section 4.6) in patients coinfected with EBV and HTLV-I [64]. Hyperinfection with *Sarcoptes scabiei* (var. *Hominis*) (Norwegian or crusted scabies) has been reported amongst Austronesians with HTLV-I [65] and in pre-ATLL [66]. Decreased delayed hypersensitivity to the purified protein derivative of tuberculosis has been repeatedly found in Japanese HTLV-I carriers [67,68]. All of these observations imply that HTLV-I has an immunosuppressive effect. It is interesting to speculate whether this may have a role in the putative synergy of HTLV-I with other oncoviruses (see Section 6.3.1.1).

***HTLV-I deleted provirus and disease.*** In a significant proportion of ATLL cases (> 30%) the clonally integrated HTLV-I provirus contains deletions with sparing of the 3' end of the virus [69]. In some HTLV-I seronegative patients with Sjögren's syndrome sequences from the *tax* gene have been found [70–72] in labial salivary glands. Rare cases of seronegative HAM/TSP with incomplete HTLV-I provirus have been reported [73].

The reported association of mycosis fungoides, a chronic T-cell cutaneous lymphoma, with HTLV p19 antigen [74], and with deleted proviral HTLV-I [75] is now thought to be spurious [76].

***Diseases associated with HTLV-II.*** Although the first two isolates of HTLV-II came from patients with hairy cell leukaemia (HCL), extensive case series have failed to identify further cases and HTLV-II is no longer thought to be associated with HCL. A number of cases of large granulocytic leukaemia [77, 78] and HTLV-II have been reported. Some patients with HTLV-II and a typical HTLV-associated myelopathy, have been described [79,80]. An ataxic variant of HAM/TSP has been reported in others [81,82]. A variety of pulmonary conditions including asthma have recently been documented among Amerindian populations in which HTLV-II infection is endemic [83].

### 6.3.2 Molecular epidemiology

The consensus view is that HTLV-I infection has been present in *Homo sapiens* for many thousands of years as a result of one or more cross-species transmissions. This is supported by phylogenetic analysis of DNA proviral sequences from the *env* gene and the long terminal repeat (LTR). *Figure 6.4* illustrates the similarity of viruses isolated from many parts of the world. The lack of diversity between these isolates suggests that HTLV-I is a stable virus evolving at a much slower rate than other RNA viruses. It is hypothesized that HTLV-I and HTLV-II may be evolving less rapidly because they are less dependent on RT for replication. This is supported by the observation that polyclonal expansion of HTLV-I-infected lymphocytes occurs in patients with HAM and in carriers [84]. Thus, at least part of the proviral burden appears to be the consequence of proliferation of infected cells and, hence, replication of proviral DNA by cellular DNA polymerase which is much more stringent than RT.

The most divergent strain, $HTLV_{MEL}$, has been found in Melanesians and Austronesians, including tribal populations who have enjoyed contact with the rest of the world only during the last 15 years. It is thought that these populations migrated to their current homes more than 7000 years ago. HTLV-I may have infected humans for 30 000 to 300 000 years. The main or cosmopolitan strain has been found throughout the world including many isolated ancient populations such as Inuits with only 4% sequence divergence between isolates. This has prompted speculation on the migration patterns of humans based on sequence analysis of HTLV-I isolates. It should also be noted that simian T-lymphotropic virus sequences cluster by region with the human sequences rather than by species.

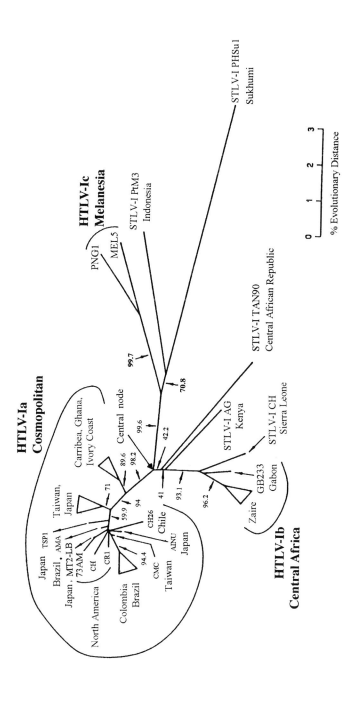

**Figure 6.4.** Unrooted phylogenetic tree of HTLV-I/STLV-I strains based on a 645 bp consensus partial LTR sequence using the neighbour-joining method. Reproduced from Liu et al. 1996, Journal of General Virology, volume 77, with permission from the Society for General Microbiology.

### 6.3.3 Seroepidemiology

*Africa.* Whether or not HTLV-I had its origins there, Africa is considered to form the largest reservoir of HTLV-I infection (*Figure 6.5*). Fleming *et al.* [107] and Hunsmann *et al.* [108] were the first to report serological evidence of HTLV-I in Africa among humans and old world monkeys. Many studies have confirmed that HTLV-I is present at a low level (< 1%) throughout western and central Africa with a seroprevalence of up to 10% in parts of Gabon [109] and Zaire [110]. HTLV-I is much less prevalent in northern and eastern Africa but is endemic in the Seychelle Islands [111–112].

*Asia and the Middle East.* The HTLV-I endemic has been most extensively documented in Japan where it is estimated that 1.2 million people are infected [121]. The infection is most common in southwest Japan including the Islands of Okinawa with a seroprevalence of up to 15% with clustering so that in some villages 30% of the inhabitants are infected. HTLV-I infection is also found in the north of Japan but is unusual in central Japan except amongst migrants from the endemic regions. The inhabitants of central Japan are thought to have migrated from mainland Asia 2300 years ago displacing the original occupants to the north and south west. It is interesting to note that the prevalence of HTLV-I in many other countries of far east Asia, including Korea [122], is low and that HTLV-I infection has not been confirmed in Siberia except on the far eastern seaboard which lies to the north of Japan [120] (*Figure 6.6*).

The Middle East is emerging as an area of HTLV-I endemicity. It has been known since 1990 that HTLV-I was prevalent amongst Jewish people from Mash-had, a region in the north of Iran [127]. More recently it has transpired that HTLV-I is also prevalent amongst the Muslim population of this region as

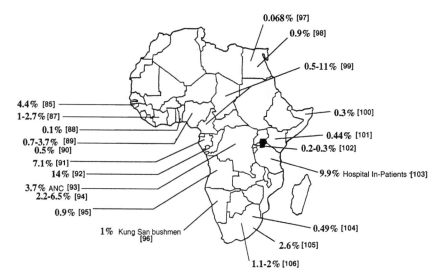

**Figure 6.5.** Seroprevalence of HTLV-I in Africa. ANC ante-natal clinic patients.

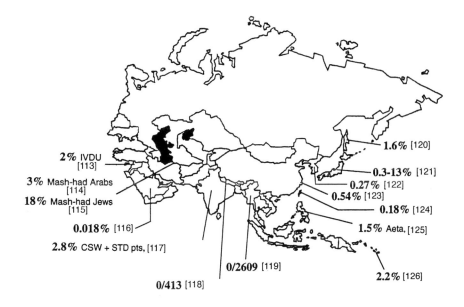

**Figure 6.6.** Seroprevalence of HTLV-I in Asia and the Middle East. IVDU, intravenous drug users; CSW, commercial sex workers; STD pts, sexually transmitted disease clinic patients.

well as in neighbouring Turkmenistan [115]. Cases of HTLV-I infection and disease have been reported from, and screening of blood donors introduced in, a number of Middle East states [116,128,129].

***The Americas.*** Movements across the Bering Straits or perhaps, approximately 12 000 years ago, the Beringia land bridge have resulted in HTLV-I being endemic amongst some Amerindians of British Columbia, Inuits and Eskimos. Further south, HTLV-I has been reported mostly amongst Afro-Americans [143]. HTLV-I is endemic in many Caribbean islands with approximately 2–5% of the population being seropositive [144–146]. South America *(Figure 6.7)* has been a 'melting pot' of races. HTLV-I has been found in a number of Amerindian peoples such as the Tumaco of Colombia whose facial appearance has prompted comparison with the Japanese and an ancient common lineage has been supported by similarities in mitochondrial DNA and human leucocyte antigen (HLA) as well as HTLV-I sequences. More recent migrations of Africans and Japanese have also brought HTLV-I infection which has been reported across the continent. Amongst Brazilian blood donors there is considerable regional variation but an estimated 0.5% are seropositive by enzyme-linked immunosorbent assay, suggesting up to 1 million infected persons in Brazil alone.

***Pacific Islands.*** Of the population of the Solomon Islands 2.2% have HTLV-I antibodies [126] including Polynesians infected with the Cosmopolitan

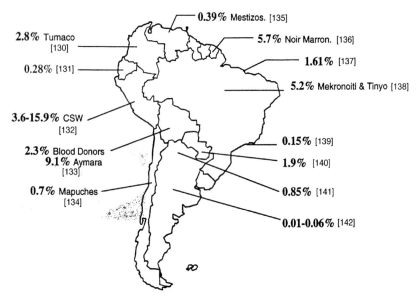

**Figure 6.7.** Seroprevalence of HTLV-I in South America. Tumaco, Aymara, Mapuches, Mekronoiti and Tinyo are tribes which reflect the indigenous population of South America. Mestizos are a mixed racial group and the Noir Marron are descendants of African slaves.

genotype and living on outlying islands. Other Polynesian populations are not infected with HTLV-I and the infection may be relatively recent. HTLV-I has not been found in all Melanesian populations e.g. Fiji but is found in a number of Austronesian populations [147–148].

***Europe.*** Western Europe cannot be considered to have any endemic regions (earlier reports from southern Italy have been refuted) but HTLV-I infection is present amongst immigrants from endemic areas and there is evidence of spread, particularly by sexual transmission from males to females, to the native European population. Amongst blood donors, a heavily preselected population, HTLV-I infection is found in 2–13 per 100 000 – many of whom are white European. Routine donor screening has been introduced nationally in France, Holland, Denmark, Sweden, Finland and Portugal. Limited data suggest a much higher seroprevalence amongst women attending antenatal clinics who are likely to be more representative of the general population. Sporadic cases have been reported where no risk for HTLV acquisition can be elicited. Although data are sparse, a seroprevalence study from Romania and case reports of ATLL in Romanians and Georgians suggest the possibility of endemic loci in central and eastern Europe [149].

***HTLV-II.*** HTLV-II has been shown to be endemic in many Amerindian populations of both north (e.g. Navajo, Pueblo and Seminole), central (Guaymi) and south (e.g. Guahibo, Kayapo and Kraho) America [150]. Until recently the only other infections were found in intravenous drug users (IVDU) in North America and Europe in whom HTLV-II is often a coinfection with HIV-1. Circumstantial and direct evidence indicate that HTLV-II was prevalent in this population before HIV-1. Thus, HTLV-II was considered to be a new world virus, until 1992 when Goubau *et al.* [151] isolated HTLV-II from central African pygmies. These findings have been confirmed by others, whereas the enticing report of HTLV-II in Mongolia [152] has yet to be confirmed and may be imported infection. HTLV-II infection is endemic amongst IVDU in Vietnam, probably a recent importation [153].

### 6.3.4 Clinical epidemiology

ATLL occurs in 2–4% of HTLV-I infected persons with little geographical or ethnic variation in frequency [25]. The disease occurs after a long incubation and infection in the perinatal period may be required for the subsequent development of ATLL. There are, however, considerable differences in prevalence of HAM/TSP in different geographical areas with the same HTLV-I seroprevalence. Thus, in Japan the prevalence of HAM/TSP in HTLV-I-positive patients is 0.003% with a calculated lifetime risk of 0.25% [154] whilst in Martinique (West Indies) the lifetime risk is 1.5–3% [155]. It is difficult to extrapolate either figure to Europe but in Brazil Caucasians, Afro-Americans and Mulattos appear to be at similar risk for developing HAM/TSP [156]. The Miyazaki cohort study has followed 525 HTLV-I seropositive carriers for 12 years during which four patients have developed ATLL but no cases of HAM have been diagnosed [157]. In a small UK prospective study out of 12 initially asymptomatic carriers followed for 2 years, one developed HAM and another HTLV-I-associated uveitis [158]. Similarly, in a survey of HTLV-I seropositive USA blood donors 2.5% had HAM/TSP at the time of first assessment [79]. This suggests that genetic or environmental co-factors may be important in the development of HTLV-I-associated inflammatory disease.

## 6.4 Evidence for oncogenesis

HTLV type I, but not type II (for which there was insufficient evidence), has been classified as an agent carcinogenic to humans (Group 1) by the International Agency for Research on Cancer, 1996 on the basis of epidemiological, animal and biological data.

### 6.4.1 Epidemiological data

Establishing the role of HTLV-I in the genesis of ATLL is dependent either on fulfilling Koch's postulates (see *Table 1.2)* or upon good epidemiological data. The first is difficult given that only a minority of subjects infected with HTLV-I develop ATLL, and then only after many years, usually decades, of infection and occasionally lymphoma/leukaemia resembling ATLL occurs in HTLV-I uninfected subjects. The epidemiological data may be supported by evidence of a similar process in other species infected with the same or a related virus and by pathogenesis and mechanistic studies which may also include experimental animal data. Animal or cellular model data alone are unlikely to provide sufficient data to implicate a virus in the oncogenic process. In the case of ATLL and HTLV-I the epidemiological data are to some extent weakened because very soon after the initial association of HTLV-I and ATLL the detection of HTLV-I, at least by serological methods, became an essential component to the diagnosis of ATLL. Indeed to be certain of the diagnosis of ATLL it is widely accepted that monoclonal (or oligoclonal) integration of HTLV-I into the genome of the malignant cell population should be demonstrated, although in practice this is usually reserved for atypical cases.

Different types of epidemiological study carry different weight in the assessment of causal association. The most reliable data come from cohort and case-control studies as from these the relative risk of developing the malignancy in those exposed (or in the case of an infectious cause, those infected) can be compared with unexposed populations.

***Cohort studies.*** Three males and two females died of ATLL among 3991 HTLV-I seropositive blood donors in Kyushu, Japan during a mean follow-up of 2.7 years [159]. In Nagasaki Prefecture two out of 503 HTLV-I seropositive patients died from ATLL compared with none out of 1494 seronegative subjects during an average follow-up of 5.3 years [160]. The diagnosis of HTLV-I was made by a particle agglutination test which is known to be very sensitive but lacks specificity. During short-term observation the risk of developing HTLV-I-associated disease appears to be small, but this may considerably underestimate the lifetime risk of developing disease. The Miyazaki cohort was established in 1984 in Miyazaki Prefecture, an area of south Japan where 26.8% of the population have antibodies to HTLV-I. The 1960 subjects comprise 70% of the population of the two villages targeted. At the time of the last published analysis the cohort had been followed for 11 years during which time 8.3% of the cohort had died, and four out of 525 (0.7%) HTLV-I seropositive subjects had developed ATLL [157]. In 1987–8, 201 seropositive and 225 seronegative subjects were enrolled in a Jamaican cohort study; at enrolment one HTLV-I-positive subject had previously undiagnosed HAM but no ATLL was diagnosed [161].

***Case-control studies.*** Whilst case series usually carry less authority than cohort studies, in the context of HTLV-I and ATLL the most convincing data are from the first case reports and case series. The T- and B-Cell Malignancy Study Group [162] reported that all 130 patients with ATLL in Kyushu were HTLV-I seropositive compared with 8% of the healthy adult population. Interestingly 24.5% of patients with non-T-cell lymphoma were also HTLV-I positive. That this may be due to blood transfusion with HTLV-I-infected blood is supported by data from other districts of Japan with a much lower (0.8%) background seroprevalence where HTLV-I infection was found in only 3.4% of patients with non-T-cell lymphoma but 90.7% of patients with ATLL [162]. Similar results have been reported from Brazil where 0.7% of the population studied were HTLV-I seropositive compared with 90.5% of ATLL patients [163]. In Trinidad and Tobago, 5.6% of healthy adults, 4% of non-T-cell lymphoma patients and 94% of patients with ATLL are infected with HTLV-I [164].

Two studies have investigated the mothers of patients with HTLV-I and shown that whilst 27–30% of the mothers of patients with HAM/TSP are also HTLV-I infected, 100% of the mothers of patients with ATLL are HTLV-I infected. This suggests that perinatal transmission of HTLV-I is important in the development of a malignancy which occurs five to six decades later [165–166].

### 6.4.2 Animal data

An early seroprevalence study of HTLV-I in Africa described the presence of antibodies in both human and non-human primates (henceforth abbreviated to primate) [108]. It is now well recognized that many African and Asian primate species are infected with a virus which has 90–95% sequence homology with HTLV-I. This has been designated simian T-cell lymphotropic virus (STLV) type-I. Phylogenetic analysis reveals clustering of STLV-I which is more dependent on geography than on species. Indeed, Asian STLV-I clades (or genotypes) cluster more closely with the Melanesian HTLV-I clade than with other STLV-I clades. In Africa the S4 clade clusters with the Zairian HTLV-I. These analyses point to several simian–human and simian–simian transmissions.

Although sometimes less detailed than human studies there have been several reports associating antibodies to HTLV-I/STLV-I with lymphoproliferative disease in a variety of primate species: 11 out of 13 macaques with lymphoproliferative disease had detectable antibodies compared with only seven out of 95 healthy macaques [167]. Similarly in a colony of 3000 baboons with a background seroprevalence of 40% all 28 baboons with lymphoproliferative disease were STLV-I-positive [168].

In the Sukhumi Primate Centre the observation that 57 out of 58 baboons with lymphoproliferative disease had antibodies to STLV-I compared with 80 out of 177 healthy baboons [169] was complicated by experiments in the 1960s when human leukaemic blood was introduced into the Centre. This was, of course, unscreened for HTLV-I. Only recently has it been demonstrated that the lymphomas in the baboons contain monoclonally integrated STLV-I of rhesus rather than of human origin [128]. T-cell lymphoproliferative disease has also been reported in an HTLV-I-infected gorilla [170] and in African green monkeys [171].

There is thus an association between STLV-I and T-cell

lymphoproliferative disease in several primate species although as in the case of humans with HTLV-I, the majority of infected subjects remain disease-free. In addition, monoclonal integration of the proviral DNA in the malignant cells is a feature of the disease, but monoclonal integration has also been detected in African green monkeys by Southern blotting in animals without disease. Sensitive techniques in humans have revealed that polyclonal expansion of HTLV-I infected CD4+ cells is a frequent occurrence in patients with HAM/TSP and in healthy carriers [84].

BLV, the other, more distant member of the family, is associated with the development of B-cell malignancy in 5% of infected cattle but 100% of experimentally infected sheep [172].

## 6.5 Transforming functions of HTLV-I

### 6.5.1 The HTLV genome

The genomes of simple retroviruses carry three genes which encode only core, polymerase and envelope proteins (Gag, Pol and Env), flanked by LTR sequences. The *Oncovirinae* and *Lentivirinae* have regulatory genes in addition to these structural genes and are termed complex retroviruses [174]. The HTLV-I genome is approximately 9 kb in length. In addition to the three standard genes an additional region, originally known as pX, houses four open reading frames which encode two regulatory proteins, Tax and Rex and three additional proteins p12, p13 and p30 (*Figure 6.8*). Rex regulates viral gene expression post-transcriptionally [175–177], while Tax is the trans-acting transcriptional activator [178–180]. In the search for the mechanism by which

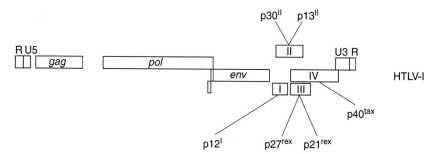

**Figure 6.8.** Schematic representation of the genomic structure of HTLV-I. The proviral genome is approximately 9 kb in length. Open reading frames (ORFs) are flanked by long terminal repeat sequences comprising direct repeats of U3 (from sequences unique to the 3' region of the genomic RNA), R (repeated at both the 5' and 3' termini) and U5 (unique to the 5' end). These sequences play a key role in transcription. Positions of the known HTLV-I genes are shown. Spaces represent non-translated regions. I, II, III, IV refer to ORFs encoding p12$^I$; p13$^{II}$ and p30$^{II}$ which are nuclear and nucleolar proteins, respectively; Rex p27 and p21 (from an alternatively spliced RNA transcript) and Tax p40. (From [173] with permission).

HTLV-I induces and/or maintains the lymphoproliferative process much attention has fallen on the product of the *tax* gene.

### 6.5.2 Tax

The Tax protein, a 42 kDa nuclear phosphoprotein, initiates transcription by activating (transcription) factors which bind to Tax-responsive elements, TRE-1 and TRE-2 located in the U3 region of the 5' LTR of the provirus. This indirect mechanism involves protein intermediaries in the form of a considerable range of cellular transcription factors which then interact with the Tax-responsive elements (*Table 6.2*). For example, TRE-1 interacts with proteins such as the cyclic AMP-responsive element (CRE) binding proteins activating transcription factor via recognition of a basic domain leucine zipper motif (bZIP) [187–190]. Tax activates transcription for both the HTLV-I LTR and the CRE-containing promoters of a variety of cellular oncogenes (among them c-*fos*, c-*myc*, c-*egr*) by binding to bZIP on one or more transactivation factors. This results in either an amplification of the transcription factor–target DNA interaction [183] or in a modification of the DNA binding specificity [191].

In addition to the CREs, Tax activates transcription following recognition of any member of the NF-κB family of transcription factors [185], the binding site for which is present in several genes with a possible role in transformation events. These include genes encoding cytokines such as granulocyte–macrophage colony stimulating factor [192] and tumour necrosis factor-β [193] as well as the IL-2Rα gene [187] encoding the Tac antigen detected in primary ATLL cells and the HIV LTR [194]. Tax interacts with NF-κB by two independent mechanisms, in the cytoplasm as well as in the nucleus. IκBα and IκBγ are proteins which inhibit NF-κB proteins by blocking their transport to the nucleus following binding in the cytoplasm. When cells are activated, IκBα and IκBγ are phosphorylated, resulting in the dissociation of the NF-κB Inhibitor complex and, thus, removal of the block on entry into the nucleus. Tax, by being able to bind to the inhibitors, forces the dissociation of the complex, increasing turnover and transport [195,196] and hence nuclear concentration of NF–κB.

A third Tax target sequence known to mediate activation of cellular immediate early genes is the serum response factor, (p67SRF) which interacts either via the CArG responsive element or directly with Tax [186].

**Table 6.2.** Cellular transcription factors which interact with HTLV-I Tax

| Factor | Reference |
|--------|-----------|
| CREB | [181,182] |
| bZIP | [183] |
| CREM | [184] |
| NFκB | [185] |
| SRF | [186] |

The alternative response element, TRE-2 harbours recognition sites for transcription factors such as Sp1, TIF-1, Ets1 and Myb [197–202].

### 6.5.3 Transformational paradigms

HTLV-I is a transforming virus but since there is no oncogene in the HTLV genome, how do these viruses effect transformation? One possible explanation is insertional mutagenesis [203], whereby the viral genome integrates into host cell chromosomal DNA adjacent to a cellular oncogene which is then activated to induce abnormal growth characteristics in the cell. The argument against this rationale is that the HTLV genome integrates in an apparently random manner [204]. Another possibility is that Tax up-regulates DNA synthesis in a less specific manner forcing the cell through its cycle without pausing in G1 to repair DNA damage. The proliferating cell nuclear antigen (PCNA) plays a key role in cell proliferation with peak PCNA mRNA levels correlating with DNA synthesis. Tax has been shown to activate the PCNA promoter which may result in an imbalance between levels of PCNA and its inhibitor [205]. Tax has also been reported to down-regulate the (β polymerase gene which encodes a protein involved in cellular DNA repair [206].

Because activation of the *tax* gene can exert an influence on the expression of other cellular genes, such as IL-2 and its cellular receptor, it may be that such activation leads to an autocrine mechanism of transformation. In other words, a situation would arise whereby an infected cell able to secrete its own growth factor could, as a result, stimulate itself to divide continuously [207]. This is difficult to demonstrate experimentally, since expression of Tax did not immortalize human lymphocytes *in vitro* [208,209], Tax expression in transgenic mice produces a benign tumour of little similarity to the natural disease [210,211] and not all ATLL cells express IL-2.

However, not only will Tax transactivate from its own promoter, but it is also able to exert an indirect influence on a number of heterologous promoters. Specific recognition by Tax of target sequences in the promoter DNA is a prerequisite for transcriptional activation of cellular genes. Some examples of these are given in *Table 6.3*. It follows that because it transactivates cellular genes which are involved in cell proliferation, Tax is likely to play a central role in the ability of HTLV-I to transform cells.

### 6.5.4 The role of Tax in transformation

**In vitro.** Primary T lymphocytes fractionated from peripheral or cord blood can be maintained in culture in conditioned medium containing IL-2 (which used to be called T-cell growth factor) [11]. Exposure of T cells to HTLV-I or HTLV-II *in vitro* induces continuous cell proliferation (immortalization) which eventually produces an IL-2-independent cell line (the process of transformation). In practice this is achieved by co-cultivating the primary target cells with mitomycin C-treated or lethally irradiated HTLV-I/II-producing cells [220,

**Table 6.3.** Cellular genes transactivated by HTLV-I Tax

| Gene | Reference |
| --- | --- |
| IL-2 | [212] |
| IL-2Rα | [207] |
| IL-3 | [213] |
| Act-2 cytokine | |
| β globulin | |
| Vimentin | |
| Class 1 MHC | |
| Granulocyte–macrophage colony stimulating factor | [192] |
| Transforming growth factor β1 | [215] |
| PtHr-P (Q46) | [216] |
| c–fos | [217] |
| c–sis | [218] |
| egr–1 | [219] |
| egr–2 | |
| PCNA | [205] |
| β–polymerase | [206] |

221]. The pivotal role of the Tax protein in this property of the human leukaemia viruses comes from experiments in which the *tax* gene transduced into recipient cells either via a retroviral vector [222] or by using a herpes virus vector [223,224], altered the growth characteristics of the cells.

Co-cultivation of peripheral blood mononuclear cells (PBMC) or cord blood lymphocytes with HTLV-producing cells most efficiently establishes transformed lines from the CD4-expressing T-cell lineage, although positive selection for CD8+ cells prior to co-cultivation can also lead to immortalization [225].

Additionally, EBV-negative HTLV-I infected B-cell lines have been reported [220,226], as well as immortalization of lymphocytes from bone marrow cell populations [227]. Nor is this property restricted to human target cells (lymphocytes from primates, rabbits, cats, mice and rats have been similarly transformed) or even to lymphocytes. Morphological changes consistent with transformation are observed on transfection of *tax* into rat embryo [228] or murine fibroblasts, the latter proving to be tumorigenic in nude mice [229]. However, information about the tumorigenic properties of *tax in vivo* has come from work using transgenic mice.

Much of the study of cell transformation by HTLV-I has come from the study of cell lines derived from ATLL patients. However, it should not be assumed that these cell lines reflect the *in vivo* situation or indeed are immortalized ATLL cell lines. As early as 1983 Hoshino [230] noted differences between ATLL cells and the HTLV-transformed cell lines. Viral antigen which usually cannot be detected by indirect immunofluorescence in fresh leukaemic cells is found following a short period of culture. ATLL cells have a single or few HTLV-I integration sites whilst the cell lines contained many integration sites [231]. The clonal nature of ATLL, recognized by the rearrangement of the

T-cell receptor (TCR) gene or by detecting the site(s) of integration of HTLV-I is regarded as a diagnostic feature of ATLL, indeed it can be used to distinguish ATLL from other T-cell leukaemias/lymphomas occurring in HTLV-I-infected carriers. However, the TCR gene rearrangements in the cell lines derived from PBMC from ATLL patients were different from the original ATLL cells [231]. Exceptional cell lines derived from patients with ATLL have been reported with identical TCR rearrangements and HTLV-I integration sites to the fresh ATLL cells [232]. Thus it appears that the majority of the HTLV-I immortalized cell lines are not the progeny of ATLL cells but may be non-malignant lymphocytes infected by HTLV-I during the early culture of ATLL cells.

**In vivo.** It has been very difficult to demonstrate viral expression, antigen or mRNA in ATLL cells or in PBMCs of healthy carriers using immunofluorescence and Southern blotting. Only by RT–PCR has *tax/rex* mRNA been detected in fresh PBMCs from patients with ATLL (five out of six) and asymptomatic carriers (four out of eight) [233]. Even with this very sensitive technique the amount of mRNA transcribed *in vivo* appears to be $10^5$–$10^6$ times less than in MT-2 cells, an HTLV-I transformed cell line. In another study HTLV-I mRNA was detected in about one in 1000 PBMCs from only two out of 15 patients with HAM/TSP [234]. Conversely, Hirose *et al.* [235] reported detecting mRNA in 1.5–7.4% of leucocytes in three ATLL patients. Using *in situ* hybridization Sonoda's group [236] has detected HTLV-I expression in fresh ATLL cells, but only in very few cells and whether the expression came from the leukaemic cells or from HTLV-I-infected non-malignant cells is not known [236].

It is therefore uncertain whether ATLL cells express HTLV-I virus or viral proteins *in vivo*. At best, it would appear that only a very small percentage of ATLL cells express HTLV-I at any time, similar to the situation in patients without malignancy. Two further observations are pertinent. Firstly, the peripheral blood of the majority of patients with asymptomatic HTLV-I infection, as well as those with HAM/TSP, contains anti-Tax-specific cytotoxic T-lymphocytes (CTL) which do not require pre-stimulation to lyse cells expressing Tax peptides [237]. Conversely, a Tax-specific CTL response is usually absent in patients with ATLL. This may be due to the immune deficiency which is a feature of ATLL or because ATLL cells do not express viral antigen, and therefore escape immune recognition. In the severe combined immune deficient (SCID) mouse model, while clones of fresh ATLL cells proliferated PBMCs and cell lines grow only when the natural killer (NK) cell activity of the mouse had also been knocked out [238]. This would infer that HTLV-I-expressing cells were killed by the NK activity and, thus, that the ATLL cells were not HTLV-I antigen expressing. Additionally, although the transplanted lymphomas grew in the SCID mice, demonstration of HTLV mRNA proved difficult. If ATLL cells do not express any HTLV-I mRNA then any role for Tax in leukaemogenesis must occur at an earlier stage of malignant transformation, or in a precursor cell not present in the peripheral blood.

Transgenic mice carrying the HTLV-I *tax* gene under the control of the virus LTR manifest a variety of symptoms, including thymic atrophy, mesenchymal tumours, epithelial cell proliferation, muscle degeneration and medullary tumours. Interestingly, no lymphoma or leukaemias develop in LTR-*tax* transgenic mice. This may be a reflection of expression levels, since LTR-*tax* is expressed to a lesser extent in lymphoid tissue than in muscle, brain, skin and salivary glands [209].

### 6.5.5 Which cell is proliferating in ATLL?

One of the paradoxes of ATLL is that the cells are mature and yet the condition is rapidly progressive. What is the evidence that the lymphocyte seen in the peripheral blood is the malignant cell? Most lymphocytes in peripheral blood in ATLL are in G0. Oligoclonal expansion of HTLV-I infected cells is a feature of HAM/TSP and healthy carriers [84] and clonal expansion is also reported in HTLV-II asymptomatic infection. The 'flower cells' which are characteristic of ATLL are also seen in up to 50% of asymptomatic carriers [158,239]. HTLV-I was absent from CD34+ cells (haematopoietic progenitor cells) in patients with ATLL [240] although these cells can be infected *in vitro* [240].

### 6.5.6 HTLV-I env is mitogenic

Tax need not be the only suspect. The HTLV-I envelope protein, gp46, is mitogenic in culture [242,243] and induces IL-2 and the IL-2 receptor (IL2-R) expression. Whilst it is likely that this phenomenon may be important in establishing infection, it is not clear whether it contributes to malignant transformation.

### 6.5.7 Tax induces apoptosis

Tax-transformed rat-1 fibroblasts undergo apoptosis following serum starvation [244]. Jurkat T cells, transiently transfected with the *tax* gene under the control of the oestrogen receptor promoter, up-regulated markers of activation after 3 days of Tax expression. In the longer term, however, proliferation was inhibited and the cells underwent apoptosis [245]. Thus, it seems that Tax expression alone may be toxic to cells and the presence of other viral or cellular proteins may be necessary to protect against apoptosis and permit transformation.

### 6.5.8 Other transforming proteins

The protein p12[I] is encoded by single- and double-spliced mRNAs transcribed from the pX region, localizes to the perinuclear compartment and the cellular endomembranes [246] and has an amino acid sequence similar to the bovine papillomavirus E5 oncoprotein (see Section 3.5.4). Both proteins are hydrophobic and contain a glutamine residue between two potential transmembrane regions. p12$^I$ can bind to the cellular target of the E5 protein, the 16K component of the vacuolar H+ ATPase protein, as efficiently as E5 and can potentiate the transforming activity of E5 in a mouse fibroblast cell line [247]. p12$^I$ has also been shown to bind to the (β and $γ_c$ chains of IL-2R [248], but the pathophysiological significance of this has not been demonstrated.

### 6.5.9 Abnormalities in tumour-suppressor genes

Abnormalities in tumour suppressor genes have been reported in ATLL but no specific or consistent abnormality has been found. Thus, in one study separate mutations in the p53 gene were found in two out of 12 patients with ATLL, one of which was associated with increased expression of p53 protein [249]. In a case study aberrant expression of p53 was reported in ATLL cells infiltrating muscle [250]. Cesarman *et al.* [251] looked for abnormalities in p53, K-*ras*, N-*ras*, H-*ras*, Rb and c-*myc* oncogenes but the only abnormalities were in p53. Mutations in p53 were found in three out of 10 cases of ATLL and were accompanied by altered p53 expression. It has been suggested that the prolonged half-life of wild-type p53, which has been demonstrated in HTLV-I transformed cell lines represents inactivation of the protein [252]. Cereseto *et al.* [253] also found evidence of impaired function of the wild-type p53 expressed in HTLV-I-transformed cells, when measuring the response to ionizing radiation and yet noted increased expression of wild-type p53 activated fragment 1/cyclin dependent kinase interacting protein 1 (p21$^{waf1/cip1}$) in all HTLV-I transformed cell lines examined. That the p53-independent expression of p21$^{waf1/cip1}$ gene is Tax-driven was suggested by observing similar expression in a Tax expressing human T-cell line [253]. p21$^{waf1/cip1}$ has been postulated to be a cyclin/cyclin dependent kinase (cdk) inhibitor which acts to block the cell cycle (see Section 3.5.3). However it has also been shown to be a component of active cyclin/cdk complexes. In addition it has been proposed that it can act as an assembly factor promoting the formation of such active complexes. In this context it may be significant that p21$^{waf1/cip1}$ is not found in resting lymphocytes but is induced following activation and proliferation [253]. Loss of the cyclin-dependent kinase-4 inhibitor (p16), which is said to be specific to lymphoid tumours, was found in five out of 14 ATLL cases [254], with deletions in 17% of acute or lymphomatous cases, but not in chronic ATLL [255]. However one patient with chronic ATLL developed deletions in p16 (and p15, another putative tumour suppressor gene) when she progressed to the acute phase. Abnormalities in these genes may therefore be associated with progression of ATLL to more aggressive forms but whether HTLV-I is implicated in this remains uncertain.

## 6.6 Treatment and prevention strategies

### *6.6.1 Treatment*

The accepted wisdom is that HTLV-I, despite lifelong infection, causes disease in fewer than 5% of carriers and that such disease occurs after several decades of infection. The development of HAM/TSP within a mean period of 3.3 years and in some cases within months of transfusion with infected blood is the recognized exception to this rule. There also appear to be some differences in prognosis for carriers in different geographical locations or perhaps of different genetic background. For example, the lifetime risk of developing HAM/TSP amongst Japanese HTLV-I carriers (0.25%) appears to be lower than elsewhere (< 7%). Although often of insidious onset, HAM/TSP can be subacute and rapidly progressive and even fatal, and causes considerable morbidity. The mean age of onset is in the fourth and fifth decades of life but the disease can present in much younger carriers resulting in decades of illness. Various treatments have been proposed, few have been subjected to placebo controlled evaluation, and the evidence of benefit is equivocal. The majority of treatments have an immunomodulatory perspective.

Adult T-cell leukaemia/lymphoma presenting with the acute or lymphomatous form is difficult to treat and, despite combination chemotherapy with regimens such as CHOP (C, cyclophosphamide; H, Doxorubicin; O, Vincristine (Oncovin); P, prednisolone) which induce partial or complete remission in the majority of patients, early relapse is common. The median survival time in 854 Japanese patients seen between 1984 and 1987 was 10 months [256]. In a recent analysis of 21 cases of ATLL presenting to two London Hospitals the mean survival from the time of diagnosis was 6 months with several patients dying within days of presentation with acute leukaemia complicated by hypercalcaemia and renal failure (Richardson, D., personal communication 1996). Two problems in particular are associated with ATLL which contribute to the poor prognosis: immunosuppression with a significant mortality from opportunistic infections which may be exacerbated by chemotherapy and expression of the multidrug resistance gene which effectively confers resistance to many cytolytic agents by increasing the rate at which they are pumped out of the cells.

As described above, the Tax protein of HTLV-I transactivates a number of intracellular genes including IL-2 and IL-2R. A feature of ATLL in all its forms is that the leukaemic cells express CD25 which is the alpha chain of IL-2R. This is expressed by activated lymphocytes (B and T cells), but is not expressed by resting normal lymphocytes. Thus, in theory, an antibody to IL-2R, anti-Tac antibody, would selectively target ATLL cells sparing the majority of non-ATLL T-cells. An autocrine hypothesis of carcinogenesis has been suggested in which Tax drives cells to proliferate by transactivating both IL-2 and IL-2R; thus, blocking IL-2R might inhibit the growth of the leukaemic cells. In the initial Phase I study of an unmodified murine anti-Tac antibody, complete remission was seen in two out of 19 patients, partial remission in four and a transient response in a seventh patient; relapse occurred in six of these seven patients [257].

Bone marrow transplantation in which the haemopoeitic system is ablated by radiotherapy and then replaced by donation from an HLA-matched donor (often a relative) has successfully cured ATLL [257]. However, many patients do not survive for long enough to be considered for bone marrow transplantation and others will not survive the period before the bone marrow is reconstituted. Eradication of HTLV-I provirus has been reported following successful bone marrow transplantation [258] but infection of the donor lymphocytes can occur [259].

### 6.6.2 Prevention

Strategies for vaccine development are considered in Chapter 7.

## 6.7 Conclusions concerning the oncogenesis of ATLL

ATLL, with rare exceptions, is characterized by a clonally expanded population of CD4+, CD25+ HTLV-I infected (and provirus integrated) lymphocytes, in which expression of HTLV-I genes (derived proteins/and mRNA ) is difficult to detect. HTLV-I transformed cell lines have an ATLL-like immunophenotype and constitutively express a number of cell activation genes. Some ATLL cells contain deleted HTLV-I provirus. Chromosomal abnormalities may be found. Whilst an autocrine phenomenon may occur, particularly early in infection, driving cell proliferation this probably does not account for the malignant transformation. ATLL occurs many decades after primary HTLV-I infection. Whilst an active anti-Tax CTL response is usually not detected in ATLL, it is common in both HAM/TSP and asymptomatic carriage and appears to reflect recent or current Tax expression. The presence of a strong CTL response and the low frequency of Tax detection even in patients with high proviral load suggests rapid clearance of Tax-expressing cells. The SCID mouse model suggests a role of NK cells in clearing Tax-expressing cells. Tax expression induces apoptosis *ex vivo* and *in vitro*. Thus, Tax expression does not seem conducive to persistence of the virus in the host. Transactivation of cellular genes, including PCNA and activation genes, and down-regulation of (β polymerase, is likely to result in a DNA mutation which may render the infected cell susceptible to malignant transformation following further 'hits'. The cell may persist in the host because it no longer expresses HTLV-I Tax or other immunoepitopes. Given the many millions of cells that may be infected during a lifetime of infection this process may occur in a small proportion of patients.

# References

1. International Committee on the Taxonomy of Viruses Sixth Report (1995).*Virus Taxonomy: Classification and Nomenclature of Viruses.* Springer-Verlag, Vienna and New York.
2. **Doolittle, R.F., Feng, D.F., McClure M.A. and Johnson M.S.** (1990) in *Retroviruses – Strategies of Replication.* (eds R. Swanstrom and P. Vogt). Springer-Verlag, New York, pp. 1–18.
3. **Piller, G.J.** (1997) *Proc. R. Coll. Physicians Edinb.* **27**(suppl.3): 1–11
4. **Ellermann, V. and Bang, O.** (1908) *Zntral. Bakteriol* **46**: 595–609.
5. **Rous, P.** (1911) *J. Exp. Med.* **13**: 397–411.
6. **Gross, L.** (1951) *Proc. Soc. Exp. Biol. Med.* **76**: 27–32.
7. **Vallee, H. and Carree, H.** (1904) *Compt. Rend. Acad. Sci.***139**: 1239–1247.
8. **Poiesz, B.J., Ruscetti, F.W., Gazdar, A.F., Bunn, P.A., Minna, J.D. and Gallo, R.C.** (1980) *Proc. Natl Acad. Sci. USA* **77**: 7415–7419.
9. **Mizutani, S., Boettige, D. and Temin, H.M.** (1970) *Nature* **228**: 424–427.
10. **Baltimore, D.** (1970) *Nature* **226**: 1209–1211.
11. **Morgan, D.A., Ruscetti, F.W. and Gallo, R.C.** (1976) *Science* **193**: 1007.
12. **Uchiyama, T., Yodoi, J., Sagawa, K., Takatsuki, K. and Uchino, H.** (1977) *Blood* **50**: 481–492.
13. **Hinuma, Y., Nagata, K., Hanaoka, M., Nakai, M., Matsumoto, T., Kinoshita, K.I., Shirakawa, S. and Miyoshi, I.** (1981) *Proc. Natl Acad. Sci. USA* **78**: 6476–6480.
14. **Seiki, M., Hattori, S., Hirayama, T. and Yoshida, M.** (1983) *Proc. Natl Acad. Sci. USA* **80**: 3618–3622.
15. **Kalyanaraman, V.S., Sarngadharan, M.G., Robert-Guroff, M., Miyoshi, I., Golde, D. and Gallo, R.C.** (1982) *Science* **218**: 571–573.
16. **Epstein, M.A., Achong, B.A. and Ball, G.** (1974) *J. Natl Cancer Inst.* **53**: 681–688.
17. **Stancek, D. and Gressnerova, M.** (1974) *Acta Virol.* **18**: 365.
18. **Cameron, K.R., Birchall, S.M. and Moses, M.A.** (1978) *Lancet* ii: 796.
19. **Muller, H.K., Ball, G., Epstein, M.A., Achong, B.G., Lenoir, G. and Levin, A.** (1980) *J. Gen. Virol.* **47**: 399–406.
20. **Loh, P.C., Mutsuuru, F. and Mizumoto, C.** (1980) *Intervirology* **13**: 87–90.
21. **Mahnke, C., Kashaiya, P., Rössler, J.** *et al.* (1992) *Arch. Virol.* **123**: 243–253.
22. **Schwiezer, M., Turek, R., Hahn, H., Schliephake, A., Netzer, K.-O., Eder, G., Reinhardt, M., Rethwilm, A. and Neumann-Haefelin, D.** (1995) *AIDS Res. Hum. Retroviruses* **11**: 161–170.
23. **Ali, M., Taylor, G.P., Pitman, R., Parker, D., Rethwilm, A., Cheingsong-Popov, R., Weber, J.N., Bieniasz, P.D., Bradley, J. and McClure, M.O.** (1996) *AIDS Res. Hum. Retrovirus* **12**: 1473–1483.
24. **Yodoi, J., Takatsuki, K. and Msuda, T.** (1974) *New Engl J. Med.* **290**: 572–573.
25. **Murphy, E.L., Hanchard, B., Figueroa, J.P., Gibbs, W.N., Lofters, W.S., Campbell, M., Goedert, J.J. and Blattner, W.A.** (1989) *Int. J. Cancer* **43**: 250–253.
26. **Chen, Y.-C., Wang, C.-H., Su, I.-J., Hu, C.Y., Chou, M.J., Lee, T.H., Lin, D.T., Chung, T.Y., Liu, C.H. and Yang, C.S.** (1989) *Blood* **74**: 388–394.
27. **Miyazaki, K., Yamaguchi, K., Tohya, T., Ohba, T., Takatsuki, K. and Okamura, H.** (1991) *Obstet. Gynecol.* **77**: 107–110.

28. Strickler, H.D., Rattray, C., Escoffery, C., Manns, A., Schiffman, M.H., Brown, C., Cranston, B., Hanchard, B., Palefsky, J.M. and Blattner, W.A. (1995) *Int. J. Cancer* **61:** 23–26.

29. Maruyama, H., Okayama, A., Kawano, T. *et al.* (1995) *J. Acquir. Immune Defic. Syndr. Hum. Retrovirol.* **10:** 262 (abstract).

30. Mueller, N., Marshall, L., Stuver, S. *et al.* (1995) *J. Acquir. Immune Defic. Syndr. Hum. Retrovirol.* **10:** 258 (abstract).

31. Greenberg, S.J., Jaffe, E.S., Ehrlich, G.D., Korman, N.J., Poiesz, B.J. and Waldman ?? (1990) *Blood* **76:** 971–976.

32. Veyssier-Belot, C., Couderc, L.J., Desgranges, C., Leblond, V., Dairou, F., Coubarrere, I. and de Gennes, J. (1990) *Lancet,* **336:** 575.

33. Penn, I. (1983) *J. Clin. Lab. Immunol.* **12:** 1–10.

34. Gessain, A., Vernant, J.C., Maurs, L., Barin, F., Gout, O., Calender, A. and de Thé, G. (1985) *Lancet* **ii:** 407–409.

35. Osame, M., Usuku, K., Izumo, S., Ijichi, N., Amitani, H., Igata, A., Matsumoto, M. and Tara, M. (1986). *Lancet* **i:** 1031–1032.

36. Osame, M., Janssen, R., Kubota, H. *et al.* (1990) *Ann. Neurol.* **28:** 50–56.

37. Gout, O., Baulac, M., Gessain, A. *et al.* (1990) *New Engl. J. Med.* **322:** 383–388.

38. Copplestone, J.A., Prentice, A.G., Hamon, M.D., Gawler, J. and Anderson, N. (1994) *Br. Med. J.* **308:** 273.

39. Mochizuki, M., Watanabe, T., Yamaguchi, K., Takatsuki, K., Yoshimura, K., Shirao, M., Nakashima, S., Mori, S., Araki, S. and Miyata, N. (1992) *Jpn. J. Cancer Res.* **83:** 236–239.

40. Mochizuki, M., Tajima, K., Watanabe, T. and Yamaguchi, K. (1994) *Br. J. Ophthalmol.* **78:** 149–154.

41. Mochizuki, M., Ono, A., Ikedo, E., Hikita, N., Watanabe, T., Yamaguchi, K., Sagawa, K. and Ito, K. (1996) *J. Acquir. Immune Defic. Syndr. Hum. Retrovirol.* **13:** S50–S56.

42. Ohba, N., Nakao, K., Isashiki, Y., Osame, M., Sonoda, S., Yashiki, S., Yamaguchi, K., Tajima, K. and the Study Group for HTLV-I Associated Ocular Disease (1994) *Jpn. J. Ophthalmol.* **38:** 162–167.

43. Merle, H., Smajda, D., Bera, O., Cabre, P. and Vernant, J.C. (1994) (in French). *J. Fr. Ophtalmol.* **17:** 403–413.

44. Nakao, K., Ohba, N., Otsuka, S., Okubo, A., Yanagita, T., Hashimoto, N. and Arimura, H. (1994) *Jpn. J Ophthalmol.* **38:** 56–61.

45. St Clair Morgan, O., Rodgers-Johnson, P., Mora, C. and Char, G. (1989) *Lancet* **ii:** 1184–1187.

46. Higuchi, I., Nerenberg, M., Yoshimine, K., Yoshida, M., Fukunaga, H., Tajima, K. and Osame, M. (1992) *Muscle Nerve* **15:** 43–47.

47. Maruyama, I., Tihara, J., Sakashita, I. *et al.* (1988) *Am. Rev. Respir. Dis.* **137:** 46.

48. Mukae, H., Kohno, S., Morikawa, N., Kadota, J., Matsukura, S. and Hara, K. (1994) *Microbiol. Immunol.* **38:** 55–62.

49. Nishioka, K., Maruyama, I., Sato, K., Kitajima, I., Nakajima, Y. and Osame, M. (1989) *Lancet* **i:** 441.

50. Kitajima, I., Maruyama, I., Maruyama, Y., Ijichi, S., Eiraku, N., Mimura, Y. and Osame, M. (1989) *Arthrit. Rheum.* **32:** 1342–1344.

51. Kitajima, I., Yamamoto, K., Sato, K., Nakajima, Y., Nakajima Y., Maruyama, I., Osame, M. and Nishioka, K. (1991) *J. Clin. Invest.* **88:** 1315–1322.

52. Ijichi, S., Matsuda, T., Maruyama, I., Izumihara, T., Kojima, K., Nimura, T., Maruyama, Y., Sonoda, S., Yoshida, A. and Osame, M. (1990) *Ann. Rheum. Dis.* **49**: 718–721.

53. Matsumoto, Y., Hibino, N., Kamimura, M. *et al.* (1990) *Jpn. J. Int. Med.* **79**: 1589–1590.

54. Eguchi, K., Matsuoka, N., Ida, H. et al. (1992) *Ann. Rheum. Dis.* **51**: 769–776.

55. Green, J.E., Hinrichs, S.H., Vogel, J. and Jay, G. (1989) *Nature* **341**: 72–74.

56. La Grenade, L., Hanchard, B., Fletcher, V., Cranston, B. and Blattner, W. (1990) *Lancet* **336**: 1345–1347.

57. LaGrenade, L., Thompson, D., Fitz-Henley, M., Dixon, J., Hanchard, B. and Manns, A. (1997) *VIIIth International Conference on Human Retrovirology;* HTLV: abstract CS20.

58. Kawai, H., Kashiwagi, S., Inui, T., Tamaki, Y., Sano, Y. and Saito, S. (1991) *J. Exp. Med.* **38**: 99–102.

59. Kawai, H., Inui, T., Kashiwagi, S., Tsuchihashi, T., Masuda, K., Kondo, A., Niki, S., Iwasa, M. and Saito, S. (1992) *J. Med. Virol.* **38**: 138–141.

60. Nakada, K., Kohakura, M., Komoda, H. and Hinuma, Y. (1984) *Lancet* i: 633.

61. Neva, F.A., Murphy, E.L., Gam, A., Hanchard, B., Figueroa, J.P. and Blattner, W.A. (1989) *New Engl. J. Med.* **320**: 252–253.

62. Nakada, K., Yamaguchi, K., Furugen. S. *et al.* (1987) *Int. J. Cancer* **40**: 145–148.

63. Patey, O., Gessain, A., Breuil, J., Courillonmallet, A., Daniel, M.T., Miclea, J.M., Roucayrol, A.M., Sigaux, F. and Lafaix, C. (1992) *AIDS* **6**: 574–579.

64. Katsuki, T., Katsuki, K., Imai, J. and Hinuma, Y. (1987) *Jpn. J. Cancer Res.* **78**: 639–642.

65. Mollison, L.C., Lo. S.T.H. and Marning, G. (1993) *Lancet* **341**: 1281–1282.

66. Daisley, C., Charles, W. and Suite, M. (1993) *Trans. R. Soc. Trop. Med. Hyg.* **87**: 295.

67. Tachibana, N., Okayama, A., Ishizaki, J., Yokota, T., Shishime, E., Mura, K., Shioiri, S., Tsuda, K., Essex, M. and Mueller, N. (1988) *Int. J. Cancer* **42**: 829–831.

68. Murai, K., Tachibana, N., Shiori, S., Shishime, E., Okayama, A., Ishizaki, J., Tsuda, K. and Mueller, N. *J. Acquir. Immune Defic. Syndr. Hum. Retrovirol.* **3**: 1006–1009.

69. Korber, B., Okayama, A., Donnelly, R., Tachibana, N. and Essex, M. (1991) *J. Virol.* **65**: 5471–5476.

70. Mariette, X., Agbalika, F. and Daniel, M.T. (1993) *Arthrit. Rheum.* **36**: 1423–1428.

71. Mariette, X., Cherot, P., Cazals, D. Brocheriou, C., Brouet, J.C. and Agbalika, F. (1995) *Lancet* **345**: 71.

72. Sumida, T., Yonaha, F., Maeda, T., Kita, Y., Iwanoto, I., Koike, T. and Yoshida, S. (1994) *Arthrit. Rheum.* **37**: 545–550.

73. Daenke, S., Parker, C.E., Niewiesk, S., Newsom-Davis, J., Nightingale, S. and Bangham, C.R. (1994) *J. Infect. Dis.* **169**: 941.

74. Turbitt, M.L. and MacKie, R.M. (1985) *Lancet* ii: 945.

75. Hall, W.W., Liu, C.R., Schneewind, O., Takahashi, H., Kaplan, M.H., Roupe, G. and Vahlne, A. (1991) *Science* **253**: 317–320.

76. Bazarbachi, A., Soriano, V., Vallejo, A., Moudgil, T., Peries, J., de Thé, H. and Gill, P.S. (1995) *Blood* **86** (suppl. 1): 928a.

77. Loughran, T.P., Coyle, T., Sherman, M.P., Starkebaum, G., Ehrlich, G.D., Ruscetti, F.W. and Poiesz, B.J. (1992) *Blood* **80**: 1116–1119.
78. Martin, M.P., Biggar, R.J., Hamlin-Green, G., Staal, S. and Mann, D. (1993) *AIDS Res. Hum. Retroviruses* **9**: 715–719.
79. Murphy, E.L., Fridey, J., Smith, J.W., Engstrom, J., Sacher, R.A., Miller, K., Gibble, J., Stevens, J., Thomson, R., Hansma, D., Kaplan, J., Khabbaz, R. and Nemo, G. (1997) *Neurology* **48**: 315–320.
80. Harrington, Jr, W.J., Sheremata, W.A., Hjelle, B., Dube, D.K., Bradshaw, P., Foung, S.K., Snodgrass, S., Toedter, G., Cabral, L. and Poiesz, B. (1993) *Ann. Neurol.* **33**: 411–414.
81. Hjelle, B., Appenzeller, O., Mills, R., Alexander, S., Torrez-Martinez, N., Jahnke, R. and Ross, G. (1992) *Lancet* **339**: 645–646.
82. Sheremata, W.A., Harrington, W.J., Bradshaw, P.A. Foung, S.K., Raffanti, S.P., Berger, J.R., Snodgrass, S., Resnick, L. and Poiesz, B.J. (1993) *Virus Res.* **29**: 71–77.
83. Giusti, R.M., Garcia, F., Stephens, K. *et al.* (1994) *AIDS Res. Hum. Retroviruses* **10**: 447.
84. Wattel, E., Cavrois M., Gessain, A. and Wain-Hobson, S. (1996) *J. Acquir. Immune Defic. Syndr. Hum. Retrovirol.* **13**(Suppl.1): S92–S99.
85. Norrgren, H., Andersson, S., Naucler, A., Dias, F., Jahansson, I. and Biberfeld, G. (1995) *J. Acquir. Immune Defic. Syndr. Hum. Retrovirol.* **9**: 422–428.
86. Liu, H.F., Goubau, P., Van-Brussel, M., Van-Laeethem, K., Chen, Y.C., Desmyter, J. and Vandamme, A.M. (1996) *J. Gen. Virol.* **77**: 359–368.
87. Ouattara, S.A., Gody, M. de Thé G. (1989) *J. Acquir. Immune Defic. Syndr. Hum. Retrovol. 189* **2**: 481–485.
88. Dumas, M., Houinato, D., Verdier, M., Zohoun, T., Jasse, R., Bonis, J., Zohoun, T., Massougbodji, A. and Denis, F. (1991) *AIDS Res. Hum. Retroviruses* **7**: 447–451.
89. Fleming, A.F., Maharajan, R., Abraham, M., Kulkarni, A.F.G., Bhusnurmath, S.R., Okpara, R.A., Williams, A.F., Akinsete, I., Schneider, J., Bayer, H. *et al.* (1986) *Int. J. Cancer* **38**: 809–813.
90. Olusanya, O., Lawoko, A. and Blomberg, J. (1990) *Scand. J. Infect. Dis.* **22**: 155–160.
91. Delaporte, E., Peeters, M., Bardy, J.L., Ville, Y., Placca, L., Bedjabaga, I., Larouze, B. and Piot, P. (1993) *AIDS Res. Hum. Retrovirol.* **6**: 424–428.
92. Goubau, P., Carton, H., Kazadi, K., Muya, K.W. and Desmyter, J. (1992) *Trans. R. Soc. Trop. Med. Hyg.* **84**: 577–579.
93. Delaporte, E., Buve, A., Nzila, N., Goeman, J., Dazza, M.C., Henzel, D., Heyward, W., St Kouis, M., Piot, P. and Laga, M. (1995) *J. Acquir. Immune Defic. Syndr. Hum. Retrovirol.* **8**: 511–515.
94. Jeannel, D., Garin, B., Kazadi, K., Singa, L, and de Thé, G. (1993) *J. Acquir. Immune Defic. Syndr. Hum. Retrovirol* **6**: 840–844.
95. Andersson, S., Dias, L., Cambelela, *et al.* (1997) VIIIth International Conference on Human Retrovirology: HTLV, Rio de Janeiro, June 9–13, abstract ED19.
96. Steele, A.D., Bos, P., Joubert, J.J., Evans, A.C., Josph, S., Tucker, L., Aspinall, S. and Lecatsas, G. (1994) *Am. J. Trop. Med. Hyg.* **51**: 460–465.
97. el Farrash, M.A., Badr, M.F., Hawas, S.A., el Nashar, N.M., Imai, J., Komoda, H. and Hinuma, Y. (1988) *Microbiol. Immunol.* **32**: 981–984.

98. Constantine, N.T., Fathi–Sheba, M., Corwin, A.L., Danahy, R.S., Callahan, J.D. and Watts, D.M. (1991) *Epidemiol. Infect.* **107**: 429–433.

99. Delaporte, E., Peeters, M., Durand, J-P., Dupont, A., Schrijvers, D., Bedjabaga, L., Honore, C., Ossari, S., Trebucq, A., Josse, R. and Merlin, M. (1989) *J. Acquir. Immune Defic. Syndr. Hum. Retrovirol.* **2**: 410–413.

100. Scott, D.A., Corwin, A.L., Constantive, N.T., Omar, M.A., Guled, A., Yusef, M., Roberts, C.R. and Watts, D.M. (1991) *Am. J. Trop. Med. Hyg.* **45**: 653–665.

101. Songok, E.M., Tukei, P.M., Libondo, D., Gichogo, A. and Oogo, S.A. (1994) *J. Acquir. Immune Defic. Syndr. Hum. Retrovirol.* **7**: 876–877.

102. Rwandan HIV Seroprevalence Study Group (1989) *Lancet* i: 941–943.

103. Schmutzhard, E., Fuchs, D., Hengster, P., Hausen, A., Hofbauer, J., Pohl, P., Rainer, J., Reibnegger, G., Tibyampansha, D., Werner, E.R. *et al.* (1989) *Am. J. Epidemiol.* **130**: 309–318.

104. Taylor, M.B., Parker, S.P., Crewe–Brown, H.H., McIntyre, J. and Cubitt, W.D. (1996) *Epidemiol. Infect.* **117**: 343–348.

105. Bhigjee, A.I., Vinsen, C., Windsor, I.M., Gouws, E., Bill. P.L. and Tait, D. (1993) *S. Afr. Med. J.* **83**: 665–667.

106. Van der Ryst, E., Joubert, G., Smith, M.S., Terblanche, M., Mollentze, F. and Pretorius, A.M. (1996) *Cent. Afr. J. Med.* **42**: 65–68.

107. Fleming, A.F., Yamamoto, N., Bhusnurmath, *et al.* (1983) *Lancet* ii: 334–335.

108. Hunsmann, G., Schneider, J., Schmitt, J. and Yamamoto, H. (1983) *Int. J. Cancer* **32**: 329–332.

109. Delaporte, E., Monplaisir, N., Louwagie, J. *et al.* (1991) *Int. J. Cancer* **49**: 373–376.

110. Goubau, P., Carton, H., Kazardi, K., Muya, K.W. and Desmyeter, J. (1990) *Trans. R. Soc. Trop. Med. Hyg.* **84**: 577–579.

111. Román, G.C., Schoenberg, B.S., Madden, D.L., Sever, J.L., Hugon, J., Ludolph, A. and Spencer, P.S. (1987) *Arch. Neurol.* **44**: 605–607.

112. Lavanchy, D., Bovet, P., Hollanda, Shamlaye, C.F., Bucezak, J.D. and Lee, H. (1991) *Lancet* **337**: 248–249.

113. Maayan, S., Dan, M., Marlink, R. and Chen, Y.M. (1992) *Int. J. Epidemiol.* **21**: 995–997.

114. Safai, B., Huang, J.L., Schutzer, P. and Ahkami, R. (1997) VIIIth International Conference on Human Retrovirology: HTLV, Rio de Janeiro, abstract MV11.

115. Achiron, A., Pinhas-Hamiel, O., Doll, L., Djaldettim, R., Chenm, A., Zivm, I., Avnim, A., Frankelm, G., Melamedmm, E. and Shohat, B. (1993) *Ann. Neurol.* **34**: 670–675.

116. Fathalla, S.E. (1997) VIIIth International Conference on Human Retrovirology: HTLV, Rio de Janeiro, abstract ED97.

117. Babu, P.G., Saraswathi, N.K., John, T.J., Ishida, T., Imai, J., Murphy, E. and Varney, K. (1992) *J. Acquir. Immune Defic. Syndr. Hum. Retrovirol.* **5**: 317.

118. Ishida, T., Takayanagi, K., Shotake, T., Hirai, K. and Yuasa, I. (1992) *Scand. J. Infect. Dis.* **24**: 399–400.

119. Burusrux, S., Urwijitaroon, Y., Romphruk, A. and Puapairoj, C. (1995) *J. Med. Assoc. Thai.* **78**: 628–630.

120. Gurtsevitch, V., Senyuta, N., Shih, J., Stepina, V., Pavlish, O., Syrtsev, A., Susova, O., Yakovleva, L., Scherbak, L. and Hayami, M. (1995) *Int. J. Cancer* **60**: 432–433.

121. Maeda, Y., Furukawa, M., Takehara, Y., Yoshimura, K., Miyamoto, K., Matsuura, T., Morishima, Y., Tajima, K., Okochi, K. and Hinuma, Y. (1984) *Int. J. Cancer* **33**: 717–720.

122. Lee, S.Y., Yamaguchi, K., Takatsuki, K., Kim, B.K., Park, S. and Lee, M. (1986) *Jpn. J. Cance. Res.* **77**: 250–254.
123. Zhuo, J., Yang, T., Zeng, Y. and Lu, L. (1995) *Chinese Med. J. Engl.* **108**: 902–906.
124. Yung, C.H., Chow, M.P., Hu, H.Y., Tzeng, J.L., Wu, Y.S., Lyou, J.S. and Liu, W.T. (1992) *Chung Hua Min Kuo Wei Sheng Wu Chi Mien I Hsueh Tsa Chih* **25**: 244–251.
125. Ishida, T., Yamamoto, K., Omoto, K. (1988) *Int. J. Epidemiol.* **17**: 625–628.
126. Yanagihara, R., Ajdukiewicz, Garruto, R.M., Sharlow, E.R., Wu, X.-Y., Alemaena, O., Sale, H., Alexander, S.S. and Gajudusek, D.C. (1991) *Am. J. Trop. Med. Hyg.* **44**: 122–130.
127. Meytes, D., Schochat, B., Lee, H., Nadel, G., Sidi, Y., Cerney, M., Swanson, P., Shaklai, M., Kilim, Y., Elgat, M. *et al.* (1990) *Lancet.* **336**: 1533–1535.
128. Voevodin, A., Al–Mufti, S., Farah, S., Khan, R. and Miura, T. (1995) *AIDS Res. Hum. Retroviruses.* **11**: 1255–1259.
129. Denic, S., Nolan, P., Doherty, J., Garson, J., Tik, P. and Tedder, R. (1990) *Lancet* **336**: 1135–1136.
130. Trujillo, J.M., Concha, M., Munoz, A., Berganzoli, G., Mora, C., Borrero, I., Gibbs, C.J. and Arango, C. (1992) *AIDS Res. Hum. Retroviruses* **8**: 651–657.
131. Cevallos, R., Barberis, L., Evans, L., Barriga, J., Verdier, M., Bonis, J., Leonard, G. and Denis, F. (1990) *J. Aquir. Immune Defic. Syndr. Hum. Retrovirol.* **4**: 1300–1301.
132. Gotuzzo, E., Sanchez, J., Escamilla, J. *et al.* (1994) *J. Infect. Dis.* **169**: 754–759.
133. Hurtado, L.V., Gomez, L.H., Andrade, R. *et al.* (1997) VIIIth International Conference on Human Retrovirology: HTLV, Rio de Janeiro, abstract ED13.
134. Inostroza, J., Diaz, P. and Saunier, C. (1991) *Scand. J. Infect. Dis.* **23**: 507–508.
135. Echeveria de Pérez, G., Loreto, O., Bianco, N.E., Mendez–Castellanos, H., Burczak, J.D. and Lee, H. (1992) *AIDS Res. Hum. Retroviruses* **8**: 219–220.
136. Tuppin, P., Lepere, J.F., Carles, G., Ureta–Vidal, A., Gerard, Y., Peneau, C., Tortevoye, P., de Thé, G., Moreau, J.P. and Gessain, A. (1995). *J. Acquir. Immune Defic. Syndr. Hum. Retrovirol.* **8**: 420–425.
137. Saraiva, J.C.P., Saraiva, A.S.L. and Couroucé, F.C.A.M. (1989) XII Congresso Nacional do Colégio Brasileiro de Hematologia, Fortaleza.
138. Nakauchi, C.M., Linhares, A.C, Maruyama. K., Kanzaki, L.I., Macedo, J.E., Azevedo, V.N and Casseb, J.S. (1990) *Mem. Inst. Oswaldo Cruz* **85**: 29–33.
139. Ferreira, O.C., Va, R.S., Carvalho, M.B., Guerra, C., Fabron, A.L., Rosemblit, J. and Hamerschlak, N. (1995) *Transfusion* **35**: 258–263.
140. Cabral, M., Vera, M.E., Cabello, A., Rios, R., Multare, S., Zapiola, I., Muchinik, G. and Bouzas, M.B. (1997) VIIIth International Conference on Human Retrovirology: HTLV, Rio de Janeiro, abstract ED41.
141. Biglione, M., Pizzaro, M., de Vito, C., Gomez, A., Serevich, I., Martinez Peralta, L., Libonatti, O. and Avila, M. (1997) VIIIth International Conference on Human Retrovirology: HTLV, Rio de Janeiro, abstract ED09.
142. Bouzas, M.B., Zapiola, I., Quiruelas, S., Gorvein, D., Panzita, A., Rey, J., Carnese, F.P., Corral, R., Perez C., Zala, C., Gallo, D., Hanson, C.V. and Muchinik, G. (1994) *AIDS Res. Hum. Retrovinises* **10**: 1567–1571.
143. Weinberg, J.B., Spiegel, R.A., Blazey, D.L., Janssen, R.S., Kaplan, J.E., Robert–Guroff, M., Popovic, M., Matthews, T.J., Haynes, B.F. and Palker, T.J. (1988) *Am. J. Med.* **85**: 51–58.

144. Murphy, E.L., Gibbs, W.N., Figueroa, J.P., Bain, B., LaGrenade, L., Cranston, B. and Blattner, W.A. (1988) *J. Acquir. Immune Defic. Syndr. Hum. Retrovirol.* **1**: 143–149.

145. Daisley, H., Charles, W., Landeau. P., Jackman, L., Batson, M. and Gomez–Adams, K. (1991) *Trop. Med. Parasitol.* **42**: 404–406.

146. Allain, J.P., Hodges, W., Einstein, M.H., Geisler, J., Neilly, C., Delaney, S., Hodges, B. and Lee, H. (1992) *J. Acquir. Immune Defic. Syndr. Hum. Retrovirol.* **5**: 1230–1236.

147. May, J.T., Stent, G. and Schnagl, R.D. (1988) *Med. J. Aust.* **149**: 104.

148. Bastian, I.B., Gardner, J., Webb, D. and Garcher, I. (1993) *J. Virol.* **67**: 843–851.

149. Taylor, G.P. (1996) *J. Acquir. Immune Defic. Syndr. Hum. Retrovirol.* **13**(suppl. 1): S8–S14.

150. Hall, W.W., Ishak, R., Zhu, S.W., Novoa, P., Eiraku, N., Takahoshi, H., Ferreira, MdC., Azevedo, V., Ishak, M.O.G., Ferreira, O.C., Monken, C. and Kurata, T. (1996) *J. Acquir. Immune Defic. Syndr. Hum. Retrovirol.* **13** (suppl. 1): S204–S214.

151. Goubau, P., Desmyter, J., Ghesquiere, J. and Kasereka, B. (1992) *Nature* **359**: 201.

152. Hall, W.W., Zhu, S.W., Horal, P., Fuuta, Y., Zagaany, G. and Vahlne, A. (1994) *AIDS Res. Hum. Retroviruses* **10**: 443.

153. Fukushima, Y., Takahashi, H., Hall, W.W. *et al.* (1995) *AIDS Res. Hum. Retroviruses* **11**: 637–645.

154. Kaplan, J.E., Osame, M., Kubota, H., Igata, I., Nishitani, H., Maeda, Y., Khabbaz, R.F. and Janssen, R.S. (1990) *J. Acquir. Immune Defic. Syndr. Hum. Retrovirol.* **3**: 1096–1101.

155. Vernant, J.C., Maurs, L., Gout, O., Buisson, G., Plumelle, Y., Neisson-Vernant, C., Monplaisir, N. and Roman, G.C. (1988) *Ann. Neurol.* **23** (suppl.): S133–S135.

156. Araújo, A.Q.-C., Afonso, C.R., Schor, D., Leite, A.C. and Andrada-Serpa, M.J. (1993) *Acta. Neurol. Scand.* **88**: 59–62.

157. Mueller, N., Okayama, A., Stuver, S. and Tachibana, N. (1996) *J. Acquir. Immune Defic. Syndr. Hum. Retrovirol.* **13**: S2–S7.

158. Taylor, G.P., Tosswill, J.H.C., Matutes, E., Daenke, S., Hall, S., Bain, B., Thomas, D., Rossor, M., Bangham, C.R.M. and Weber, J.N. (submitted).

159. Tokudome, S., Maeda, Y., Fukada, K., Teshima, D., Asakura, T., Sueoka, E., Motomura, Y., Kusumoto, Y., Inamura, Y., Kiyokawa, T., Ikeda, M. and Tokunago, O. (1991) *Cancer Causes Control* **2**: 75–78.

160. Iwata, K., Ho, S.-I., Saito, H., Ito, M., Nagatomo, M., Yamasaki, T., Yoshida, S., Suto, H. and Tajima, K. (1994) *Jpn. J. Cancer Res.* **85**: 231–237.

161. Murphy, E.L., Wilks, R., Owen, St-C.M., Hanchard, B., Cranston, B., Figueroa, J.P., Gibbs, W.N., Murphy, J. and Blattner, W.A. (1996) *Int. J. Epidemiol.* **25**: 1090–1097.

162. T- and B-cell Malignancy Study Group (1985) *Jpn. J. Clin. Oncol.* **15**: 517–535.

163. Pombo de Oliviera, M.S., Matutes, E., Schultz, T., Carvalho, S.M., Noronh, H., Reaves, J.D., Loureiro, P., Machado, C. and Catovsky, D. (1995) *Int. J. Cancer* **60**: 823–827.

164. Manns, A., Cleghorn, F.R., Falk, R.T., Hanchard, B., Jaffe, J.S., Bartholomew, C., Hartge, P., Benichou, J., Blattner, W.A. and the HTLV Lymphoma Study Group. *Lancet* **342**: 1447–1458.

165. Bartholomew, C., Edwards, J., Jack, N., Corbin, D., Murphy, J., Cleghorn, F., White, F. and Blattner, W. (1994) *AIDS Res. Hum. Retroviruses* **10**: 470.
166. Wilks, R., Hanchard, B., Morgan, O., Williams, E., Cranstan, B., Smith, M.L., Rogers-Johnson, P. and Manns, A. (1996) *Int. J. Cancer* **65**: 272–273.
167. Homma, T., Kanki, P.J., King, Jr, N.W., Hunt, R.D., O'Connell, M.J., Letvin, N.L., Daniel, M.D., Desrosiers, R.C., Yang, C.J. and Essex, M.C. (1984) *Science* **225**: 716–718.
168. Hubbard, G.B., Moné, J.P., Allan, J.S., Davis, K.J., III., Leland, M.M., Banks, P.M. and Smir, B. (1993) *Lab. Anim. Sci.* **43**: 301–309.
169. Voevodin, A.F., Lapin, B.A., Yakovleva, L.A., Ponomaryeva, T.I., Oranyan, T.E. and Razmadza, E.N. (1985) *Int. J. Cancer* **36**: 579–584.
170. Srivastava, B.I.S., Wong-Staal, F. and Getchell, J.P. (1986) *Cancer Res.* **46**: 4756–4758.
171. Sakakibara, I., Sugimoto, Y., Sasagawa, A., Honjo, S., Tsujimoto, H., Nakamura, H. and Hayami, M. (1986) *J. Med. Primatol.* **15**: 311–318.
172. Dijilali, S., Parodi, A.-L., Levy, D. and Cockerell, G.L. (1987) *Leukaemia* **1**: 777–781.
173. Franchini, G. (1995) *Blood* **86**: 3619–3639.
174. Cullen, B.R. (1991) *J.Virol.* **65**:1053–1056.
175. Kiyokawa, T., Seiki, M., Iwashita, S., Imagawa, K., Shimizu, F. and Yoshida, M. (1985) *Proc. Natl. Acad. Sci. USA* **82**: 8359–8363.
176. Hidaka, M., Inoue, J., Yoshida, M. and Seiki, M. (1988) *EMBO J.* **7**: 519–523.
177. Inoue, J.-I., Seiki, M., Tanaguchi, T., Tsuru, S. and Yoshida, M. (1991) *Oncogene* **6**: 1753–1757.
178. Sodroski, J.G., Rosen, C.A. and Haseltine, W.A. (1984) *Science* **225**: 381–385.
179. Cann, A.J., Rosenblatt, J.D., Wachsman, W., Shah, N.P. and Chen, I.S.Y. (1985) *Nature* **318**: 571–574.
180. Felber, B.K., Paskalis, H., Kleinman-Ewing, C., Wong-Staal, F. and Pavlakis, G.N. (1985) *Science* **229**: 675–679.
181. Chrivia, J.C., Kwok, R.P., Lamb, N., Hagiwara, M., Montminy, M.R. and Goodman, R.H. (1993) *Nature* **365**: 855–859.
182. Kwok, R.P., Laurance, M.E., Lundblad, J.R., Goldman, P.S., Shih, H., Connor, L.M., Marriott., S.J. and Goodman, R.H. (1996) *Nature* **380**: 642–646.
183. Baranger, A.M., Palmer, C.R. Hamm, M.K., Giebler, H.A., Brauweiler, A., Nyborg, J.K. and Schepartz, A. (1995) *Nature* **376**: 606–608.
184. Zhao, L.-J. and Giam, C.-Z. (1992) *Proc. Natl. Acad. Sci. USA* **89**: 7070–7074.
185. Suzuki, T., Hirai, H. and Yoshida, M. (1994) *Oncogene* **9**: 3099–3105.
186. Fujii, M., Tsuchiya, H., Chuhjo, T., Akizawa, T. and Seiki, M. (1992) *Genes Dev.* **6**: 2066–2076.
187. Jeang, K.-T., Boros, I., Brady, J., Radonovich, M. and Khoury, G. (1988) *J. Virol.* **62**: 4499–4509.
188. Willems, L., Kettmann, R., Chen, G., Portetelle, D., Burny, A., Mammerickx, M. and Derse D. (1992) *J. Virol.* **66**: 766–772.
189. Suzuki, T., Fujisawa, J.-I., Toita, M. and Yoshida, M. (1993) *Proc. Natl. Acad. Sci. USA* **90**: 610–614.
190. Adam, E., Kerkhofs, P., Mammerickx, M., Kettmann, R., Burny, A., Droogmans, L. and Willems, L. (1994) *J. Virol.* **68**: 5845–5853.
191. Paca-Uccaralertkun, S., Zhao, L.-J., Adya, N., Cross, J.V., Cullen, B.R., Boros, I.M. and Giam, C.-Z. (1994) *Mol. Cell. Biol.* **14**: 456–462.

192. Miyatake, S., Seiki, M., DeWaal, Malefijt, R. *et al.* (1988) *Nucleic. Acids Res.* **16**: 6547–6566.
193. Paul, N.L., Millet, I. and Ruddle, N.H. (1993) *Cytokine* **5**: 372–378.
194. Jeang, K.-T., Shank, P.R. and Kumar, A. (1988) *Proc. Natl. Acad. Sci. USA*, **85**: 8291–8295.
195. Hirai, H., Suzuki, T., Fujisawa, J.I., Inoue, J.I. and Yoshida, M. (1994) *Proc. Natl. Acad. Sci. USA.* **91**: 3584–3588.
196. Suzuki, T., Hirai, H., Murakami, T. and Yoshida, M. (1995) *Oncogene* **10**: 1199–1207.
197. Bosselut, R., Duvall, J.F., Gegonne, A., Bailly, M., Hemar, A., Brady, J. and Ghysdael, J. (1990) *EMBO J.* **9**: 3137–3144.
198. Bosselut, R., Lim, F., Romond, P.-C., Frampton, J., Brady, J. and Ghysdael, J. (1992) *Virology* **186**: 764–769.
199. Gitlin, S.D., Bosselut, R., Gegonne, A., Ghysdael, J. and Brady, J.N. (1991) *J. Virol.* **65**: 5513–5523.
200. Gitlin, S.D., Dittmer, J., Reid, R.L. and Brady, J.N. (1993) in *Frontiers in Molecular Biology.* (ed B. Cullen). Oxford University Press, Oxford. pp. 159–192.
201. Yoshida, M. (1994) *AIDS Res. Hum. Retroviruses* **10**: 1193–1197.
202. Franchini, G., Tartaglia, J., Markham, P., Benson, J., Fullen, J., Wills, M. Arp, J., Dekaban, G., Paoletti, E. and Gallo, R.C. (1995) *AIDS Res. Hum. Retroviruses* **11**: 307–313.
203. Haward *et al* (1981) *Mutat. Res.*, **86** (3): 307–327.
204. Yoshida, M., Seiki, N., Yamaguchi, K. and Takatsuki, K. (1984) *Proc. Natl Acad. Sci. USA* **81**: 2534–2537.
205. Ressler, S., Morris, G.F. and Marriott, S.J. (1997) *J. Virol.* **71**: 1181–1190.
206. Jeang, K.-T., Widen, S.G., Semmes, O.J. and Wilson, S.H. (1990) *Science* **247**: 1082–1084.
207. Inoue, J.-I., Seiki, M., Tanaguchi, T., Tsuru, S. and Yoshida, M. (1986) *EMBO J.* **5**: 2883–2888.
208. Nerenberg, M., Minor, T., Price, J., Ernst, D.N., Shinohara, T. and Schwarz, H. (1991) *J. Virol.* **65**: 3349–3353.
209. Bieberich, C.J., King, C.M., Tinkle, B.T. and Jay, G. (1993) *Virology* **196**: 309–318.
210. Nerenberg, M., Hinrichs, S.H., Reynolds, R.K., Khoory, G. and Jay, G. (1987) *Science* **237**: 1324–1325.
211. Hinrichs, S.H., Nerenberg, M., Reynolds, R.K., Khoury, G., and Jay, G. (1987) *Science* **237**: 1340–1343.
212. Siekewitz, M., Josephs, S.F., Dukovich, M., Peffer, N., Wong-Staal, F. and Greene, W.C. (1987) *Science* **238**: 1575–1578.
213. Wolin, M., Kornuc, M., Hong, C., Shin, S.K., Lee, F., Lau, R. and Nimer, S. (1993) *Oncogene* **8**: 1905–1911.
214. Green, J.E. (1991) *Mol. Cell. Biol* **11**: 4635–4641.
215. Kim, S.-J., Kehrl, J.H., Burton, J. *et al.* (1990) *J. Exp. Med.* **172**: 121–129.
216. Watanabe, T., Yamaguchi, K., Takatsuki, K., Osame, M. and Yoshida, M. (1990) *J. Exp. Med.* **172**: 759–765.
217. Fujii, M., Sassaone-Corsi, P. and Verma, I.M. (1988) *Proc. Natl. Acad. Sci. USA* **85**: 8526–8530.
218. Pantazis, P., Sariban, E., Bohan, C.A., Antoniades, H.N. and Kalyanaraman, V.S. (1987) *Oncogene* **1**: 285–289.
219. Fujii, M., Niki, T., Mori, T. *et al.* (1991) *Oncogene* **6** (6): 1023–1029.

220. Yamamoto, N., Okada M., Koyanagi Y., Kannagi, M. and Hinuma, Y. (1982) *Science* **217**: 737–739.
221. Popovic, M., Lange-Wantzin, G., Sarin, P.S., Mann, D. and Gallo, R.C. (1982) *Proc. Natl. Acad. Sci. USA* **80**: 5402–5406.
222. Akagi, T. and Shimotohno, K. (1993) *J. Virol.* **67**: 1211–1217.
223. Grassmann, R., Dengler, C., Müller-Fleckenstein, I., Fleckenstein, B., McGuire K., Dokhelar, M.-C., Sodroski, J.G. and Haseltine, W.A. (1989) *Proc. Natl. Acad .Sci. USA* **86**: 3351–3355.
224. Grassmann, R., Berchtold, S., Radant, I., Alt, M., Fleckenstein, B., Sodroski, J.G., Haseltine, W.A. and Ramstdet, U. (1992) *J. Virol.* **66**: 4570–4575.
225. Sugamura, K., Sakitani, M. and Hinuma, Y. (1984) *J. Immunol. Methods* **73**: 379–385.
226. Longo, D.L., Gelmann, E.P., Cossmanm J., Young, R.A., Gallo, R.C., O'Brien, S.J., and Matis, L.A. (1984) *Nature* **310**: 505–506.
227. Markham, P.D., Salahuddin, S.Z., Macchi, B., Robert-Guroff, M., and Gallo, R.C. (1984) *Int. J. Cancer* **33**: 13–17.
228. Pozzati, R., Vogel, J. and Jay, G. (1990) *Mol. Cell. Biol.* **10**: 413–417.
229. Tanaka, A., Takahashi, C., Yamaoka, S., Nosaka, T., Maki, M. and Hatanaka, M. (1990) *Proc. Natl Acad. Sci. USA* **87**: 1071–1075.
230. Hoshino, H., Esumi, H., Miwa, *et al.* (1983) *Proc. Natl. Acad. Sci. USA* **80**: 6061–6065.
231. Maeda, H., Shimizu, A., Ikuta, K., Okamoto, H., Kashihara, M., Uchiyam, T., Honjo, T. and Yodoi, J. (1985) *J. Exp. Med.* **162**: 2169–2174.
232. Yamada, Y., Nagata, Y., Kamihira, S., Tagawa, M., Ichimaru, M., Tomonaga, M. and Shiku, H. (1991) *Leuk. Res.* **15**: 619–625.
233. Kinoshita, T., Shimoyama, M., Tobinai, K., Ito, M., Ito, S., Ikeda, S., Tajima, K., Shimotohno, K., Sugimura, T. (1989) *Proc. Natl. Acad. Sci. USA* **86**: 5620–5624.
234. Beilke, M.A., In, D.R., Gravell, M., Hamilton, R.S., Mora, C.A., Leon-Monzon, M., Rodgers-Johnson. P.E., Gajdusek, D.C., Gibbs, Jr, C.J., and Zaninovic, V. (1991) *J. Med. Virol.* **33**: 64–71.
235. Hirose, S. *et al.* (1992) (In Japanese). *Rinsho–Ketsueki.* **33**: 311–316.
236. Setoyama, M., Fujiyoshi, T., Mizoguchi, S., Katahira, Y., Yashiki, S., Tara, M., Kanzaki, T. and Sonoda, S. (1994) *Int. J. Cancer* **57**: 760–764.
237. Daenke, S., Kermonde, A., Hall, S.E., Taylor, G., Weber, J., Nightingale, S. and Bangham, C.R.M. (1996) *Virology* **217**: 139–146.
238. Feuer, G., Stewart, S.A., Baird, S. Lee, F., Feuer, R. and Chen, I.S.Y. (1995) *J. Virol.* **69**: 1328–1333.
239. Matutes, E., Dalgleish, A.G., Weiss, R.A., Joseph, A.P. and Catovsky, D. (1986) *Int. J. Cancer* **38**: 41–45.
240. Nagafuji, K., Harada, M., Teshima, T., Eto, T., Takamatsu, Y., Okamura, T., Murakawa, M., Akashi, K. and Niho, Y. (1993) *Blood* **82**: 2823–2828.
241. Feuer, G., Shah, N.P., Li, Q., An, D.-S., Zack, J.A. and Chen, I.S.Y. (1997) VIIIth International Conference on Human Retrovirology: HTLV, Rio de Janeiro, abstract 133.
242. Gazzolo, L. and Dodon, M.D. (1987) *Nature* **326**: 714–717.
243. Zack, J.A., Cann, A.J., Lugo, J.P. and Chen, I.S. (1988) *Science* **240**: 1026–1029.
244. Yamada, T., Yamaoka, S., Goto, T., Nakai, M., Tsujimoto, Y. and Hatanaka, M. (1994) *J. Virol.* **68**: 3374–3379.

245. Chichlia, K., Moldenhauer, G., Daniel, P.T., Busslinger, M., Gazzolo, L., Schirrmacher, V. and Khazaie, K. (1995) *Oncogene* **10**: 269–277.
246. Koralnik, I.J., Fullen, J. and Franchini, G. (1993) *J. Virol.* **67**: 2360–2366.
247. Franchini, G., Mulloy, J.C., Koralnik, I.J., Lo-Monico, A., Sparkowski, J.J., Andresson, T., Goldstein, D.J. and Schlegel, R. (1993) *J. Virol.* **67**: 7701–7704.
248. Mulloy, J.C., Crownley, R.W., Fullen, J., Leonard, W.J. and Franchini, G. (1996) *J. Virol.* **70**: 3599–3605.
249. Nagai, H., Kinoshita, T., Imamura, J. *et al.* (1991) *Jpn. J. Cancer Res.* **82**: 1421–1427.
250. Higuchi, I., Hashimoto, K., Kashio, N., Izumo, S., Matsuola, H., Nakagawa, M. and Osame, M. (1995) *Acta Neuropathol.* **90**: 323–327.
251. Cesarman, E., Chadburn, A., Inghirami, G., Gaidano, G. and Knowles, D.M. (1992) *Blood* **80**: 3205–3216.
252. Reid, R.L., Lindholm, P.F., Mireskandari, A., Dittmer, J. and Brady, J.N. (1993) *Oncogene* **8**: 3029–3036.
253. Cereseto, A., Diella, F., Nulloy, J.C., Cara, A., Michieli, P., Grassmann, R., Franchini, G. and Klotman, M.E. (1996) *Blood* **88**: 1551–1560.
254. Ogawa, S., Hangaish, A., Hirosawa, S. *et al.* (1995) *Blood* **86**: 1548–1556.
255. Hatta, Y., Hirama, T., Miller, C.W., Yamada, Y., Tomonaga, M. and Keoffler, H.P. (1995) *Blood* **85**: 2699–2704.
256. Lymphoma Study Group (1991) *Leukaemia Res.* **15**: 81–90.
257. Waldmann, T.A., White, J.D., Goldman, C.K. *et al.* (1993) *Blood* **82**: 1701–1712.
258. Borg, A., Yin, J.A., Johnson, P.R., Tosswill, J., Saunders, M. and Morris, D. (1996) *Br. J. Haematol.* **94**: 713–715.
259. Ljungman, P., Lawler, M., Asjo, B., Bogdanovic, G., Karlsson, K., Malm, C., McCann, S.R., Ringden, O. and Gahrton, G.. (1994) *Br. J. Haematol.* **88**: 403–405.

Chapter 7

# Vaccination and virus-mediated therapy

**John R. Arrand, David R. Harper, Tim J. Harrison, Myra McClure, Nicola A. Smith, Simon J. Talbot, Graham P. Taylor and Denise Whitby**

## 7.1 Introduction

The genesis of a cancer is a multifactorial process (see Sections 1.3, 2.7, 3.6 and 4.9). Different types of cancer vary in their geographical distribution presumably due to the variation in prevalence of the components of the oncogenic cocktail, be they genetic or environmental, in different parts of the world. Often the precise nature of the factors required is not clear, thus making preventive measures impracticable. In other instances, for example cigarette smoking, addictive social habits require a difficult behavioural change for a large proportion of the population in order that the reduction in associated disease may be achieved. However the inclusion of an infectious agent, a virus, as a necessary component of the oncogenic cocktail presents a real opportunity to develop effective preventative or therapeutic measures by means of vaccination against that agent.

As an example of the potential of anti-virus vaccination in terms of cancer prevention, statistics from Hong Kong (*Figure 7.1*) suggest that vaccination against Epstein–Barr virus (EBV; associated with nasopharyngeal cancer), hepatitis B virus (HBV; associated with liver cancer) and human papillomavirus (HPV; associated with cancer of the cervix) could have a beneficial effect on around 25% and 20% of cancers in males and females, respectively, in that part of the world.

Vigorous efforts are currently being made to address this issue. Vaccines against HBV are already in widespread use, several trials of HPV vaccines are

*Viruses and Human Cancer*, edited by J.R. Arrand and D.R. Harper
© 1998 BIOS Scientific Publishers Ltd, Oxford

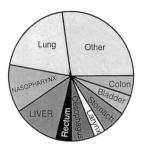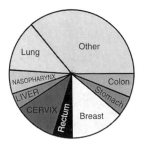

**Figure 7.1**. Relative proportions of the commonest cancers of males (left) and females (right) in Hong Kong. Virus-associated cancers are shaded. Data from [1].

in progress whilst a trial of a potential EBV vaccine has begun and others are at an advanced stage of planning.

## 7.2 Hepatitis B vaccines

### 7.2.1 Introduction

It is estimated that around 300 million individuals worldwide are carriers of hepatitis B surface antigen (HBsAg) and more than 1 million deaths each year are attributable to the sequelae of chronic HBV infection including primary liver cancer. There was a clear need for safe and effective HBV vaccines and strategies for prevention, especially for the infants of carrier mothers who may be infected perinatally, and which would result in a dramatic reduction of this toll.

Individuals who recover from acute hepatitis B produce antibodies (anti-HBs) to HBsAg and have lifelong immunity to re-infection. It was logical, therefore, to determine whether prophylactic immunization with HBsAg would elicit a protective immune response. First generation vaccines, comprising HBsAg from the donated plasma of hepatitis B carriers, are still in use in some countries. Second generation vaccines contain recombinant HBsAg synthesized in eukaryotic (yeast or mammalian) cells. Both are safe and effective.

There are minor problems with these vaccines. Up to 5% of immunocompetent recipients, especially the elderly, fail to make an antibody response. Infants of infectious mothers may become infected, sometimes despite a seemingly adequate antibody response, and viral variants which seem to escape neutralization have been isolated in some cases. Nonetheless, implementation of universal programmes of immunization should make a major impact on the prevalence of HBV infection, especially in regions where HBsAg carriage is common. The absence of an animal reservoir makes the eventual eradication of HBV possible but lifelong persistent infection and the difficulties in preventing all cases of maternal–infant transmission necessitate a programme spanning several generations.

### 7.2.2 Plasma-derived vaccines

The lack of a cell culture system for HBV necessitated the use of another source of antigen for vaccine production. The huge reservoir of HBsAg in the carrier population constituted a potential source of antigen and led to an entirely novel approach. HBV-infected hepatocytes secrete HBsAg in the form of non-infectious, subviral particles (22 nm spheres and tubules) in vast excess over the 42 nm virions. Procedures for purification and adjuvantation of HBsAg, which included several steps which would inactivate HBV and other pathogens, were developed by several manufacturers (*Figure 7.2*).

The resulting preparation was shown to be safe and immunogenic in volunteers. Furthermore, the vaccine protected chimpanzees against challenge with HBV, including cross-protection against challenge with a different subtype of the virus (e.g. *adw* vaccine and *ayw* virus) [2]. Immunization regimens were investigated and a schedule of 0-, 1- and 6-month doses was found to be quite effective. The third (booster) dose is important in increasing the seroconversion rate in immunocompetent adults from 75–85% to over 90% and in increasing the geometric mean titre of antibody [3].

The vaccine was shown to be effective in protecting recipients against

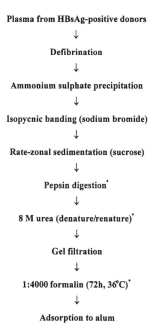

**Plasma from HBsAg-positive donors**
↓
**Defibrination**
↓
**Ammonium sulphate precipitation**
↓
**Isopycnic banding (sodium bromide)**
↓
**Rate-zonal sedimentation (sucrose)**
↓
**Pepsin digestion**[*]
↓
**8 M urea (denature/renature)**[*]
↓
**Gel filtration**
↓
**1:4000 formalin (72h, 36°C)**[*]
↓
**Adsorption to alum**

**Figure 7.2.** Typical production process for a plasma-derived hepatitis B virus vaccine. Steps marked * will inactivate viruses which may be present in donated plasma.

infection, most notably in a trial amongst high-risk individuals in New York. The vaccine will also prevent perinatal transmission from viraemic mothers to their infants, especially if the first dose is given within 24 h of birth. However, protective efficacy rates vary widely (from 70% to over 90%) and in many programmes hepatitis B immune globulin (HBIG) is administered at the same time as the first dose of vaccine (but at a different site) in order to neutralize virus from the mother. There is some evidence that high doses of vaccine may preclude the need for HBIG [4,5].

The advent of the human immune deficiency virus (HIV) pandemic, and particularly the occurrence of cases of acquired immune deficiency sydrome (AIDS) amongst the pool of donors of HBsAg-positive plasma, caused concern over the safety of first generation vaccines. Despite the fact that these concerns were unjustified and that the vaccine was perfectly safe, newly available sources of HBsAg produced using recombinant DNA technology made possible a move away from plasma-derived vaccines, particularly in the west. Plasma-derived vaccines remain an option, particularly in areas where carrier rates are high, providing that safety and quality control measures are adhered to strictly.

### 7.2.3 Recombinant vaccines

The molecular cloning of the HBV genome in the late 1970s was followed by the development of expression systems for HBsAg in yeast (*Saccharomyces cerevisiae*) and mammalian (Chinese hamster ovary, CHO) cells. Yeast systems give rather higher yields and are used more commonly. Recombinant plasmids are based on the self-replicating element, the 2 μ circle, and an expression cassette comprising the surface gene driven by a strong yeast promoter (GAL1 or PHO5) and yeast transcriptional termination sequences. Most encode only the 226 amino acid major surface protein but inclusion of pre-S2 and pre-S1 sequences (see *Figure 2.2*) is possible (see below).

HBsAg synthesized in mammalian cells is secreted into the culture fluid as 22 nm particles which resemble those found in the circulation of carriers. The protein is not secreted from yeast but particles may be detected when the cells are disrupted. An example of a purification process for a yeast-derived recombinant hepatitis B vaccine is shown in *Figure 7.3*. Yeast-derived vaccines which lack pre-S components are roughly equivalent to plasma-derived vaccines in terms of immunogenicity and protective efficacy.

Anti-HBs responses to plasma-derived and currently licensed recombinant vaccines are directed primarily to the *a* determinant of HBsAg. Most of the 226 amino acid major surface protein is hydrophobic and predicted to span the lipid bilayer of the envelope or to be internal in the virion and subviral particles (*Figure 7.4*). The immunodominant *a* determinant has been mapped to a hydrophilic region encompassing amino acids 124–147. The region is rich in cysteine residues and disulphide bridges maintain its structure, perhaps as a double loop, on the surface of the particles. The amino acid sequence, partic-

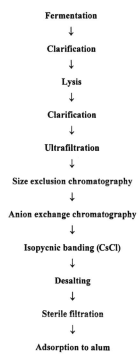

Fermentation
↓
Clarification
↓
Lysis
↓
Clarification
↓
Ultrafiltration
↓
Size exclusion chromatography
↓
Anion exchange chromatography
↓
Isopycnic banding (CsCl)
↓
Desalting
↓
Sterile filtration
↓
Adsorption to alum

**Figure 7.3.** Production process for a licensed, yeast-derived hepatitis B virus vaccine.

ularly of the 'second loop' (residues 139–147) is highly conserved among wild-type isolates of HBV and substitutions of conserved amino acids have been implicated in escape from neutralization by antibody (see Section 7.1.5).

### 7.2.4 Problems of non-responsiveness

HBV vaccines are recommended for intramuscular injection. Injection into the buttock is not recommended because deposition into fat reduces responsiveness. Because of the relatively high cost of HBV vaccines, some workers have investigated the efficacy of schedules involving lower dose intradermal injections. At least two such studies concluded that response rates and geometric mean titre of antibody were lower in subjects injected intradermally compared with those receiving intramuscular doses of vaccine [7].

As noted above, up to 5% of immunocompetent individuals fail to respond to a full course of vaccine, booster doses or a further full course may induce seroconversion in around 40% of these non-responders. Such non-responsiveness seems to increase with age. Poorer responses may be found in the immunosuppressed, including HIV-infected patients, and patients with renal failure. Studies in mice suggest that the immune responses to the major surface protein and pre-S domains are regulated separately and pre-S2 epitopes may augment the response to the major surface protein [8]. This begs the question

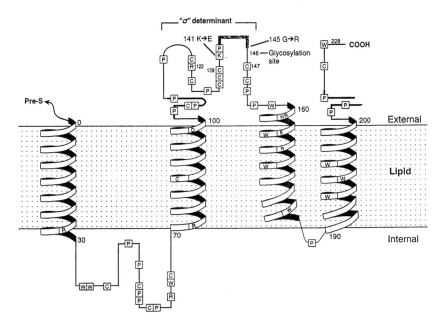

**Figure 7.4.** Proposed structure of the major hepatitis B virus surface protein showing the location of some antibody escape substititions (residues 141 and 145). Amino acid residues are denoted by the single letter code. Modified from [6].

whether inclusion of pre-S epitopes in vaccine preparations will reduce the rate of non-responsiveness (see Section 7.2.6).

### 7.2.5 Problems of vaccine failure

Protection of the infants of carrier mothers is a major challenge especially because there is a high probability that those infected perinatally will become carriers and sources of further transmission. As noted above, protective efficacy rates of over 90% may be achieved when the first dose of vaccine is administered within 12 h of birth and combined with HBIG or as part of a high dose schedule. It is important to determine why some infants become infected despite such schedules.

In some cases, infants infected perinatally despite combined immunoprophylaxis are seropositive for HBsAg and anti-HBs. Sequence analysis of HBV from such cases frequently reveals point mutations leading to unusual amino acid substitutions in the *a* determinant. The mutation observed most commonly leads to a change of the highly conserved glycine to an arginine at residue 145 of the major surface protein. Such variants have been observed in immunized subjects in Italy [9], Singapore [10], Japan [11,12] and elsewhere. In the Singapore study, variants were found in 16 out of 41 breakthrough infections and the Arg-145 substitution in 12 of these cases [13]. Other mutations which have been observed include Leu-133 [13], Glu-141 [14] and Ala-144 [15].

Most of these cases have been associated with administration of HBIG which may have selected the variant(s) from the infecting dose from the mother. In at least one case, emergence of a variant was documented in a mother several years after she infected her child. A similar situation is seen in liver transplant patients whose grafts become reinfected despite administration of anti-HBs [16]. However, in some cases the variants seem to have been selected without the administration of HBIG, for example in the Gambian study where the Glu-141 variant has been detected in the adult carrier population also.

In the case of the Arg-145 variant, it has been possible to demonstrate altered antigenic reactivity of the surface protein [17] and this is likely for the other variants. Thus far, secondary spread of the variants has not been documented but horizontal transmission remains a possibility, including to individuals who are anti-HBs-positive following immunization. It is feasible to modify vaccines to include the most common variant(s) but this is not indicated at the present time.

The majority of breakthrough infections in the Singapore study were associated with apparently wild-type virus [13]. These infants usually were HBsAg-positive at birth and remained so thereafter. HBV normally does not cross the placenta but may do so in a small percentage of cases [18]. Another study in The Netherlands correlated vaccine failure with high levels of maternal viraemia rather than non-responsiveness of the infants and concluded that transplacental transmission was responsible [19]. New strategies will be needed for the protection of such infants if HBV is to be completely eradicated.

### 7.2.6 Pre-S vaccines

Inclusion of pre-S epitopes in vaccine preparations may solve some of the problems of non-responsiveness described above. It is possible that additional epitopes would diminish pressure on the *a* determinant leading to vaccine escape mutations also. Most current vaccines do not contain pre-S epitopes. The proteolytic treatment in the production process for plasma-derived vaccine described in *Figure 7.2* removed the pre-S domains from middle and large surface proteins. Other processes which did not include this procedure resulted in plasma-derived vaccines with a variable content of pre-S proteins [20]. Most recombinant vaccines contain only the major surface protein. However, a vaccine produced in France from CHO cells includes pre-S2 proteins [21]. Disappointingly, the results from trials with pre-S2-containing vaccines suggest that non-responsiveness occurs as frequently as with vaccines containing only the major surface protein.

The pre-S1 domain of HBsAg contains an assembly signal which inhibits the secretion of the middle and major proteins from mammalian cells. It seems also to be over-glycosylated when expressed in yeast. Despite these problems, candidate pre-S1 vaccines have been produced. Early data from clinical trials suggest that these vaccines may solve some problems of non-responsiveness, particularly in the elderly [22,23].

### 7.2.7 Strategies for immunization

Many countries with a high prevalence of HBV infection have adopted pro-grammes of universal immunization of infants already. In cases where the mother is HBsAg-positive it is essential that the first dose of vaccine is given as early as possible, certainly within 12 h of birth. The use of high dose sched-ules in such cases may render administration of HBIG unnecessary and obvi-ate the need for testing the mother for viraemia (HBeAg positivity).

Many countries with a low prevalence of infection opted for a strategy of immunizing high-risk individuals only. Whilst it is essential that such individ-uals continue to be immunized, such strategies have not resulted in a decrease in the annual incidence of acute hepatitis B [24]. The World Health Organisation had recommended that universal immunization should be in place in areas with a prevalence of HBsAg greater than 8% by 1994 and in all countries by 1997. Despite failure to achieve these targets in many countries, universal immunization against HBV remains an important goal.

### 7.2.8 Universal immunization against HBV reduces the incidence of liver cancer

Several decades will be required before the full impact of HBV immunization on the incidence of primary liver cancer can be assessed. However, there already is a clear indication that the nationwide HBV vaccination programme implemented in Taiwan in July 1984 has led to a reduction in childhood liver cancer. The average annual incidence of hepatocellular carcinoma (HCC) in children 6–14 years of age declined from 0.70 per 100 000 children between 1981 and 1986 to 0.57 per 100 000 children between 1986 and 1990, and to 0.36 per 100 000 children between 1990 and 1994 [25]. The corresponding rates of mortality from HCC also decreased. The incidence of HCC in children 6–9 years of age declined from 0.52 per 100 000 children for those born between 1974 and 1984 to 0.13 per 100 000 children for those born between 1984 and 1986. There is every reason to believe that the impact on lifelong liver cancer rates will be as great.

## 7.3 Towards a hepatitis C vaccine

Several years have passed since the first reports of the discovery of hepatitis C virus (HCV) as the major causative agent of parenterally-transmitted non-A, non-B hepatitis [26,27], but a vaccine still seems a long way off. As with HBV, chronic carriers of HCV make antibodies to a variety of virus-specified pro-teins including the structural nucleocapsid protein and various non-structural proteins (see *Figure 2.4*). However, in the case of HCV, persistently infected individuals may also be seropositive for antibodies against the surface glyco-proteins of the virion [28].

Will prior immunization with viral structural proteins, particularly the surface glycoproteins, protect the naive individual against future challenge? Retrospective studies of chimpanzees used for transmission studies of non-A, non-B hepatitis, now known to be HCV, demonstrate that repeated acute infections may occur in one individual [29]. A further potential problem is that the amino terminus of the surface glycoprotein E2 (gp70), which may be a major antigenic domain on the virion surface, is highly variable [28,30]. Indeed, there is evidence that peaks of viraemia in chronically infected patients may follow the emergence of variants with mutations in the RNA encoding this region and which escape neutralization by antibody [28,30].

An efficient and reliable cell culture system for the growth of HCV has not been reported, precluding (for the time being) this route to an inactivated, whole virus vaccine. Similarly, the scarcity of suitable primate hosts and lack of markers of virulence and attenuation limit the prospects for a live, attenuated vaccine. The most straightforward approach seems to be to develop a vaccine based on HCV proteins expressed by recombinant DNA technology.

Choo *et al.* [31] expressed the surface glycoproteins of the prototype strain of HCV in cultured human cells using recombinant vaccinia virus. The viral proteins accumulated in the endoplasmic reticulum and were purified and used to immunize seven chimpanzees. Five animals were protected against challenge with live virus; the two poorest responders, in terms of antibody levels, had short, resolving acute infections. However, a number of criticisms may be made of this study. The challenge dose was low, 10 $CID_{50}$, (chimpanzee infectious $dose_{50}$, i.e. the dose which, if given to each of a group of chimpanzees, should be sufficient to infect 50% of them) and given when the antibody response was high, only 2 weeks after the final immunizing dose. Perhaps more importantly, the challenge virus was the same strain as that used for immunization. Thus, the major potential problem of variability of the surface glycoproteins was circumvented. It remains to be determined whether a cocktail of antigens might protect against a variety of HCV strains.

An alternative approach might be to immunize with a protein with less sequence variability, such as the nucleocapsid protein. Chronic infection with HCV is associated with positivity for antibodies against this protein but an immune response prior to infection might be protective, particularly if cellular as well as antibody responses were stimulated. The approach has been attempted with HBV [32,33]. Chimpanzees which were challenged with HBV following immunization with the core antigen made antibodies to the surface protein HBsAg, a phenomenon interpreted to indicate recovery from a short and mild acute infection. An HCV vaccine which protects against chronic infection may be preferable to no HCV vaccine, even if a mild and anicteric (without jaundice) acute infection ensues in the event of exposure.

Who would be the recipients of an HCV vaccine? Potential candidates include haemophiliacs, dialysis patients and the spouses of infectious individuals; the list is reminiscent of that used in the early days of HBV immunization. Yet, this targeting of high risk groups has failed to reduce the incidence of acute hepatitis B in countries such as the USA [24]. The risk of infection for the recipients of blood and blood products has diminished considerably since the introduction of donor testing programmes and inactivation procedures for blood products. The risks of sexual transmission [34] and transmission to hospital personnel [35] also seem low. The routes of transmission implicated in most sporadic cases of hepatitis C remain obscure. Until a vaccine is available which is not only safe and effective but also cheap enough for widespread application, measures such as universal precautions which prevent parenteral spread are likely to be the only way of limiting transmission of HCV.

## 7.4 Human papillomavirus vaccines

### 7.4.1 Introduction

Studies on the worldwide incidence of cervical carcinoma estimate around 460 000 new cases every year. In some parts of the world, such as China, Latin America and the Caribbean it is the commonest female cancer and on a global basis it is the second most common female cancer, after breast cancer. Given the compelling evidence of the association between the 'high-risk' human papillomaviruses (HPVs) and the development of cervical carcinoma (Chapter 3) an effective anti-HPV vaccine would be expected to have a remarkable impact on worldwide health.

Experimental work towards this goal has been concentrated mainly within two areas:(i) immunology of oncoproteins; and (ii) animal model systems.

### 7.4.2 Immunology of oncoproteins

The products of the E6 and E7 open reading frames (ORFs) of the cervical cancer-associated HPV-16 have been implicated in transformation by several independent criteria: the E6 and E7 ORFs tend to be retained and expressed in cervical tumours and in cell lines derived from them and the ORFs have demonstrable *in vitro* transforming abilities. Furthermore, it has been shown that cervical carcinoma cell lines grown in long-term culture continue to rely on E6 and E7 expression for growth. These observations suggested that immune responses, in particular cytotoxic T cells (CTL), raised against the E6 and/or E7 proteins may form the basis of potential vaccines.

### 7.4.3 Cell-mediated immunity

Several lines of evidence point to the importance of cell-mediated immune responses in the control of papillomavirus infection. Immunosuppressed patients, individuals with immunodeficiencies involving cell-mediated immunity and patients carrying HIV all exhibit enhanced papilloma proliferation and an increased frequency of HPV infection. Renal transplant recipients on long-term therapeutic immunosuppression have an increased incidence of cervical intraepithelial neoplasia lesions and HPV infections in general as compared with the normal population. In addition, regressing warts show several features characteristic of a cell-mediated immune reaction.

Cytotoxic T cells recognize foreign antigens in a human leukocyte antigen (HLA)-restricted fashion. Peptide fragments of the foreign protein are presented at the cell surface by class I HLA molecules and different HLA molecules present different fragments. Peptides are specifically bound in a groove in the HLA molecule. Analysis of such peptides shows that they are usually nine amino acids in length and contain particular, conserved amino acid residues, called anchors, at specific points (e.g. peptides which bind to HLA-B27 contain an arginine at position 2). The side chains of the anchor residues are frequently inserted into pockets within the groove of the HLA molecule where they bind via hydrophobic interaction or hydrogen bonding.

Viral proteins present in the cellular cytoplasm are degraded by proteosomes giving a mixture of peptide fragments which are transported to the endoplasmic reticulum by two transporter proteins known as TAP1 and TAP2. Here, peptides of optimal length and specificity bind to the groove of nascent HLA heavy chain or to newly formed heavy chain–β2 microglobulin complex. These complexes are then transported to the cell surface via the Golgi apparatus where glycosylation is completed. These cell surface complexes are the targets for CD8+ CTL. This scheme is shown diagrammatically in *Figure 7.5*.

Mutant cell lines which are defective in processing express empty HLA molecules at the cell surface. These empty molecules are unstable but can be stabilized by exogenous addition of appropriate peptide thereby leading to a measurable, increased level of HLA on the cell surface. One such mutant cell line is the human HLA-A2.1 line known as T2. For a more detailed discussion of antigen presentation and processing see [36,37].

This mechanism of antigen processing leads to the concept of vaccination with CTL target peptides which should in turn stimulate the generation of the appropriate population of CTL and confer protection from infection or elimination of cells expressing the appropriate viral protein. This concept has been validated in, for example, Sendai virus infection of mice where it was known that a single Sendai virus nucleoprotein peptide epitope was recognized by CTL. Following vaccination with a peptide containing this epitope the mice were protected from a five-fold lethal dose of Sendai virus [38].

Thus considerable effort has been expended in the identification of potential CTL targets within the E6 and E7 ORFs of HPV-16. A set of 240 overlapping, nonameric peptides with an eight amino acid overlap was synthesized. These peptides encompassed the entire coding sequences of the HPV-16 E6 and E7. Using the T2 mutant cell line (see above) a number of peptides have been identified which will bind to HLA-A0201, the commonest human HLA class I molecule [39].

In an alternative approach, human HLA-A0201 cells were infected with recombinant vaccinia virus expressing HPV-16 E6 or with parental, non-recombinant vaccinia. HLA molecules were isolated from the infected cells, bound peptides eluted and fractionated by high performance liquid

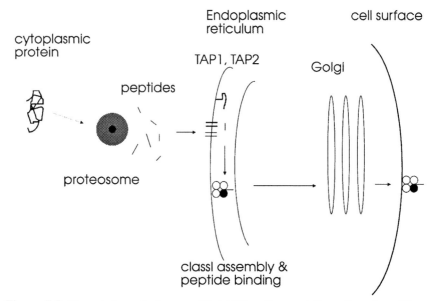

**Figure 7.5.** Presentation of virus-specified CTL epitopes at the cell surface. Virus-coded proteins are degraded by proteosomes to yield peptide fragments. These peptides are transported to the lumen of the endoplasmic reticulum via the TAP1, TAP2 transporter. Specific peptides then bind to HLA class I heavy chain, along with $\beta$-2 microglobulin. This stable complex is then further processed in the Golgi apparatus to give the mature glycosylated form, and is then transported to the cell surface.

chromatography. The peptide profiles from the E6-positive and control samples were compared and peptides which were unique to the E6-positive samples were sequenced. One peptide was identified which corresponded to E6 and thus was a naturally processed potential CTL epitope [40]. This peptide corresponded to one of those identified using the T2 binding assay. Thus a number of potential CTL target epitopes have been identified which could form the basis of immunological intervention against HPV-16-positive cervical cancer cells. Clinical trials are in progress (see Section 6.4.6).

### 7.4.4 Animal model systems

A great deal of important experimental vaccine work has been carried out using the bovine model system [41]. Cattle are susceptible to infection by a variety of bovine papillomavirus (BPV) types, two of which, BPV-2 and BPV-4, have provided the focus for vaccine development work. BPV-2 usually infects the skin causing warts, whereas BPV-4 infects the mucosa of the upper alimentary tract leading to the development of papillomas. These are most often benign and self-limiting but in animals which ingest bracken fern as part of their diet the papillomas tend to progress to cancers. This is another example of the multifactorial nature of a virus-associated cancer. Because of their tissue tropism BPV-2 and BPV-4 may be considered as models for cutaneous (e.g. HPV5) and mucosal (e.g. HPV-16 and HPV-18) human papillomaviruses, respectively.

Early experiments showed that vaccination of calves with purified virus or with virus-containing cell extracts conferred protection against further infection whereas vaccination with extracts of transformed cells which express the early gene products but not virus structural proteins were ineffective. These results together with the observation that protection correlated with the presence of neutralizing antibodies in the serum of the protected animals suggested that the virion structural proteins were responsible for the generation of the protective response.

In order to confirm this, the BPV-2 structural proteins L1 and L2 were expressed in bacteria and used separately in challenge experiments. In the case of L1 all the vaccinated animals developed neutralizing antibodies and were resistant to challenge by virus. In contrast, all of the non-vaccinated control animals developed lesions within 4 weeks of challenge. A similar effect has been observed in rabbits vaccinated with the L1 protein of cottontail rabbit papillomavirus (CRPV) and subsequently challenged with CRPV.

In contrast, vaccination of calves with L2 did not prevent the development of warts within 4 weeks of challenge. However, these warts soon became infiltrated with T cells and regressed around 10 weeks post challenge. This indicates that BPV-2 L2 elicits a cell-mediated immune response but although the vaccinated animals possessed high-titre serum antibodies against L2, these sera were not virus-neutralizing. However, similar experiments with the L2 proteins from both BPV-4 and CRPV gave rise to virus-neutralizing antibody and in the case of BPV-4 L2, this was accompanied by almost complete protection from virus challenge. In addition, the protective effect was of long duration, conferring protection for at least 1 year after vaccination.

As mentioned above, it has been argued that the transforming proteins E6 and E7 may be good targets for cell-mediated immunity. With this in mind a group of calves were vaccinated with bacterially produced BPV-4 E7 as a fusion protein with glutathione-S-transferase (GST) followed by challenge with BPV-4. Although the number of papillomas which developed was the same in both vaccinated and control animals, tumour development was inhibited in the vaccinated group and regression was more rapid than in the control group. Thus, although immunization with E7 is ineffective in prophylaxis it does appear to have a therapeutic effect.

In a rodent model, immunization with a putative high affinity CTL epitope peptide or with recombinant vaccinia viruses expressing either HPV-16 E6 or E7 conferred protection against transplanted syngeneic tumour cells that had been transfected with either the HPV-16 E7 gene or with the whole viral genome. This protective effect was mediated by CD8+ cytotoxic T cells [42, 43,44]. Although several investigators have demonstrated that HPV-specific CTL can be produced in mice, identification of the corresponding cells in humans remains elusive.

### *7.4.5 Neutralizing antibodies*

It is frequently argued that generation of neutralizing antibody response is a necessary component of a prophylactic vaccine. Although the bovine model gave encouraging results using the capsid proteins of BPV, this was not the case in some other experimental situations where purified capsid proteins were used in their non-native conformation. It has been demonstrated that conformational epitopes on intact virions induce high titres of neutralizing antibodies and confer strong protection against subsequent virus challenge [45].

A method of synthetically mimicking the surface topography of the virion is afforded by high level expression of the virion proteins in various expression systems whereby the products self-assemble to form virus-like particles (VLPs). Baculovirus and yeast expression systems have been used most commonly. In some cases L1 alone will form VLPs whereas in other situations both L1 and L2 have been found to be necessary. On injection into animals these particles generate high titre neutralizing antibodies which are type-specific, indicating that HPV virions are antigenically distinct from one another [46, 47].

Immunization of rabbits with CRPV L1 VLPs rendered the rabbits completely immune to subsequent challenge [48]. That this approach could potentially be applied to genital HPV infection is suggested by studies of a similar immunization of dogs and subsequent challenge with canine oral papillomavirus demonstrating that intradermal injection was also capable of protecting against infection at mucosal surfaces [49].

VLPs appear to be attractive candidates as vaccines; however, before they can be considered seriously, methods will need to be devised for their large-scale production and to achieve consistency between batches.

### *7.4.6 Clinical trials*

Using the results from the bovine model as a precedent, a Phase 1/Phase 2 physician-sponsored clinical trial of an HPV-16 E7–GST fusion protein has been initiated in Brisbane, Australia as a potential therapy for advanced cervical carcinoma.

A clinical trial has been initiated in Holland using a mixture of two high affinity HLA-A0201 binding peptides from HPV-16 E7 together with a synthetic helper peptide. The peptides are adjuvanted with a new type of defined adjuvant called Montanide ISA51. The trial aims to test the vaccine on cervical carcinoma patients who have not responded to conventional radiotherapy, chemotherapy and surgery, who have an HLA-A0201 tissue type and whose tumours are associated with HPV-16. Such patients would have a life expectancy of approximately 6 months. The vaccinees are being given a course of four immunizations after which CTL memory will be assayed. Ethical considerations dictate that the initial Phase 1 trials are carried out in this 'worst case' scenario. Any beneficial immunotherapeutic effect will be a very welcome bonus.

In Cardiff, Wales, a trial using a different strategy was initiated in January 1994 [50]. Eight patients, seven of whom had recurrent disease, were recruited and given a single vaccination with a recombinant vaccinia virus which expresses fusion proteins between the E6 and E7 genes of both HPV-16 and HPV-18. For safety reasons the E7 portions of the proteins have been mutated to inactivate the retinoblastoma protein binding site. The HPV status of the subjects was not determined prior to vaccination but it has subsequently been shown that seven out of the eight carry HPV-16. The recombinant was derived from the Wyeth vaccine strain of vaccinia and is attenuated with respect to the parental Wyeth virus. The recombinant is stable and following vaccination all patients exhibited conventional scabbing and an absence of systemic virus shedding. Although the vaccinees had all previously received radiotherapy and chemotherapy they all responded with a serological antibody response to vaccinia. In addition, two patients who initially had anti-E6 antibodies exhibited an increased anti-E6 titre whilst two others developed a new anti-E7 response. Two out of the four patients developed class I-restricted CTL responses as assayed using recombinant adenovirus to present the target antigen whereas four patients who were HLA-A0201 positive did not show a CTL response against the target peptides which are the subject of the Dutch trial.

Since VLPs are structurally and immunologically the same as the authentic virion they represent extremely attractive candidates for the basis of safe vaccines [51] and are currently being taken forward for clinical trials.

### 7.4.7 Potential difficulties

A complication pertaining to the concept of therapeutic intervention via induction of HPV-specific CTL (e.g. by peptide vaccination) is the observation that expression of HLA molecules is down-regulated or abolished in a significant proportion of cervical carcinomas [52]. Thus presentation of the appropriate target peptides will be compromized with resulting impairment of target cell recognition by CTL.

Second, HPV may have evolved to escape immune surveillance by mutation of CTL epitopes. An examination of the sequence of the HPV-16 E6 coding region within DNA from cervical carcinoma patients of HLA-B7 haplotype showed that 32% of the samples contained a mutation within a potential HLA-B7 restricted CTL epitope in E6. This mutation was not seen in DNA from cervical cancers in patients of differing HLA haplotypes [53]. This observation is similar to that noted for the HLA A11-restricted epitope within EBNA3b of EBV (see Section 4.6.1).

However, if peptide vaccination does prove to be effective, in addition to the problems posed by HLA polymorphism in relation to the number of epitopes required to obtain complete population-based protection, one is also faced with the multiplicity of cervical carcinoma-associated HPVs. Although initially the majority of cases potentially could be dealt with by targeting HPV-

16 and HPV-18, there are several other types, (e.g. 31, 33, 35, 39, 45, 51, 52, 56), which may fill the niche if the prevalence of the more common types is reduced. Therefore a cocktail containing a very large number of different peptides may be required in order to achieve complete cover.

## 7.5 Epstein–Barr virus vaccines

### 7.5.1 Introduction

As described in Chapter 4 EBV is associated with a wide range of acute, chronic and malignant diseases. Indeed it was the virus' associations with various human cancers which formed the prime considerations behind the call for an EBV vaccine, first proposed by Epstein in the 1970s [54]. Clearly the worldwide number of cases of EBV-associated diseases is very large and consequently a vaccine to prevent conditions induced by this agent would have a significant effect on worldwide morbidity and mortality. Despite persistent scepticism, the concept has continued to be promoted vigorously with the result that several different potential strategies for vaccination have been and continue to be explored [55]. Initial human trials are just beginning.

### 7.5.2 EBV membrane antigen

As with HCV (see Section 7.3) cell culture methods have not yet been devised which produce whole EBV in significant amounts. Therefore the classical vaccination approach of inoculating the vaccinee with an attenuated strain of the organism against which protection is sought is not applicable and for this reason the subunit vaccine concept has been adopted.

Until recently virtually all efforts towards the development of an EBV vaccine had concentrated on a subunit vaccine based on the virus membrane antigen (MA). This can be detected on the envelopes of intact virions and on the plasma membrane of virus producer cell lines and consists of at least three glycoproteins of molecular weights 340–350 kDa (gp340), 220–270 kDa (gp220) and about 85 kDa (gp85). The first two glycoproteins are the major components of MA and were shown to share antigenic determinants, a property which was subsequently demonstrated to be due to their structural relationship. The two proteins are derived from a single gene by splicing, without a change in reading frame (*Figure 7.6*). Antibodies raised against the plasma membranes of EBV-producer cell lines or EBV envelopes have virus-neutralizing activity. In addition, monoclonal antibodies or monospecific antisera which recognize EBV MA will also neutralize the virus. These data suggested that gp340/220 would form a good basis for the development of an anti-EBV vaccine.

The efficacy of the response to a vaccine immunogen is clearly influenced by antigenic variation within the target protein (see Sections 4.4, 4.6, 7.2.5,

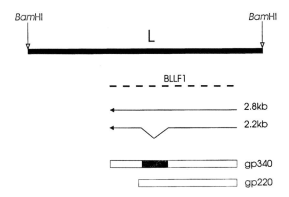

**Figure 7.6.** Relationship of gp340 and gp220. The *Bam*HI-L fragment of EBV is depicted by the line at the top (see Figure 4.2 for the complete *Bam*HI restriction map of EBV DNA). Beneath this is shown the position of the BLLF1 open reading frame within *Bam*HI-L. BLLF1 is transcribed to give two mRNAs (arrows), one of which is spliced. The unspliced transcript encodes gp340 (indicated by the box at the bottom), the spliced transcript encodes gp220 which is lacking the repeated region (shown by the shading).

7.4.7). Because, to date, all potential MA-based EBV vaccines had been derived from gp340/220 of the B95-8 A-type strain, there existed the possibility that if the glycoproteins were antigenically distinct, a B-type virus (see Section 4.4) may evade the effects of such a vaccine. Nucleotide sequence analysis of several type-A and type-B viruses and comparison with the prototype B95-8 EBV strain (type A) showed that all gp340 genes exhibited a very high degree of amino acid identity with B95-8. The sequence comparison is shown in *Figure 7.7.*

In order to determine whether this high degree of sequence homology was conserved at a functional level, a panel of 14 different monoclonal antibodies raised against A-type EBV and representing six different epitope groups along the length of the gp340 molecule was used in immunofluorescence assays against homologous A-type B95-8 cells and heterologous B-type C2.BL16 cells. It was found that all six epitope groups were recognized in both cell lines indicating functional conservation of B-cell epitopes between gp340 from both types of EBV [56]. The high degree of structural and functional homology suggests that a vaccine produced using gp340 from an A-type strain should be equally effective against type B strains.

### 7.5.3 Recombinant live virus delivery systems

Early work showed that vaccination of cottontop tamarins with gp340/220 which had been purified from B95-8 cells would prevent the establishment of massive, fatal lymphomas following challenge with a tumorigenic dose of EBV [57]. This established the principle that, at least in the tamarin

```
B95-8   MEAALLVCQY TIQSLIHLTG EDPGFFNVEI PEFPFYPTCN VCTADVNVTI NFDVGGKKHQ LDLDFGQLTP
NL      .......... .......... .......... .......... .......... .......... ..........
M81     .......... .......... .......... .......... .......... .......... ..........
AG876   .......... ......Q..R D......... L......A.. .......A.. .........K .N...L...
MT4     .......... .......... .......... .......... .......... .......... ..........

B95-8   HTKAVYQPRG AFGGSENATN LFLLELLGAG ELALTMRSKK LPINVTTGEE QQVSLESVDV YFQDVFGTMW
NL      .......... .......... .......... .......... .......... .......... ..........
M81     .......... .......... .......... .......... .......... .......... ..........
Ag876   .......... .......... .......... .......... ......I... .......... ..........
MT4     R......... .......... .......... .......... .......... .......... ..........

B95-8   CHHAEMQNPV YLIPETVPYI KWDNCNSTNI TAVVRAQGLD VTLPLSLPTS AQDSNFSVKT EMLGNEIDIE
NL      .......... .......... .......... .......... .......... .......... ..........
M81     .......... .......... .......... .......... .......... .......... Q.........
Ag876   .......... .......... .......... .......... .......... .......... ..........
MT4     .......... .......... .......... .......... .......... .......... Q.........

B95-8   CIMEDGEISQ VLPGDNKFNI TCSGYESHVP SGGILTSTSP VATPIPGTGY AYSLRLTPRP VSRFLGNNSI
NL      .......... .......... .......... .......... .......... .......... ..........
M81     .......... .......... .......... .......... .......... .......... ..........
Ag876   .......... .......... .......... .......... .......... .......... ..........
MT4     .......... .......... .......... .......... .......... .......... ..........

B95-8   LYVFYSGNGP KASGGDYCIQ SNIVFSDEIP ASQDMPTNTT DITYVGDNAT YSVPMVTSED ANSPNVTVTA
NL      .......... .......... .......... .......... .......... .......... ..........
M81     .......... .......... .......... .......... .......... .......... ..........
Ag876   .......... .......... .......... .......... .......... .......... ..........
MT4     .......... .......... .......... .......... .......... .......... ..........

B95-8   FWAWPNNTET DFKCKWTLTS GTPSGCENIS GAFASNRTFD ITVSGLGTAP KTLIITRTAT NATTTTHKVI
NL      .......... .......... .......... .......... .......... .......... ..........
M81     .......... .......... .......... .......... .......... .......... ..........
Ag876   .......... .......... .......... .......... .......... .......... ..........
MT4     .......... .......... .......... .......... .......... .......... ..........

B95-8   FSKAPESTTT SPTLNTTGFA DPNTTTGLPS STHVPTNLTA PASTGPTVST ADVTSPTPAG TTSGASPVTP
NL      .......... .......... .......... .......... .......... .......... ..........
M81     .......... .......... .......... .......... .......... .......... ..........
Ag876   .......... .......... A......... .......... .......... .......... ..........
MT4     .........S ...... .......... .......... .......... .......... ..........

                    [
B95-8   SPSPWDNGTE SKAPDMTSST SPVTTPTPNA TSPTPAVTTP TPNATSPTPA VTTPTPNATS PTLGKTSPTS
NL      .......... .......P. PA........ .......... .......... .......... ..........
M81     .......... ......**** ********** ....S..... ...G...... M......... ..........
Ag876   ....R..... ......**** ********** ....S..... .......... .......... ..........
MT4     .......... ......**** ********** ..T.L..... ......T... .......... ..........

B95-8   AVTTPTPNAT SPTLGKTSPT SAVTTPTPNA TSPTLGKTSP TSAVTTPTPN ATGPTVGETS PQANATNHTL
NL      .......... ......**** ********** *******... .......... ..S....... ..........
M81     .........* ********** ********** *******... .P........ .......... ..........
Ag876   .........* ******.... P......... .I........ .......... ..S....... ....T.....
MT4     .........* ******.... P......... .......... .......... .......... ..........

                                                                                  ]
B95-8   GGTSPTPVVT SQPKNATSAV TTGQHNITSS STSSMSLRPS SNPETLSPST SDNSTSHMPL LTSAHPTGGE
NL      .......... .......... .......... .......... .......... .......... ..........
M81     .......... .P......D. ......R... .......... .I...***** ****...... ..........
Ag876   ...S...... .P........ .......... .......... .IS....... .......... ..........
MT4     ...F...... .P........ .......... .......... .I........ .......... ..........

B95-8   NITQVTPASI STHHVSTSSP APRPGTTSQA SGPGNSSTST KPGEVNVTKG TPPQNATSPQ APSGQKTAVP
NL      .......... .......... .......... .......... .......... .......... ..........
M81     .......... .......... .......... .......... .......... ...K...... ..........
Ag876   .........T .......... .......... .......... .......... ...K...... ...\..._...
MT4     .........T .......... .......... .......... .......... ...K...... ..........

B95-8   TVTSTGGKAN STTGGKHTTG HGARTSTEPT TDYGGDSTTP RPRYNATTYL PPSTSSKLRP RWTFTSPPVT
NL      .......... .......... .......... .......... .......... .......... ..........
M81     .......... .......... .......... ......D.... .......... .......... ..........
Ag876   .......... .......... .......... .......... .T........ .......... ..........
MT4     .......... .......... .......... .......... .......... .......... ......E...

B95-8   TAQATVPVPP TSQPRFSNLS MLVLQWASLA VLTLLLLLVM ADCAFRRNLS TSHTYTTPPY DDAETYV...
NL      .......... .......... .......... .......... .......... .......... ..........
M81     .......... .......... .......... .......... .......... .......... ..........
Ag876   .......... .......... .......... .......... .......... .......... ..........
MT4     .......... .......... .......... .......... .......... .......... ..........
```

**Figure 7.7.** Comparison of the predicted gp340/220 amino acid sequences from various EBV strains. B95-8, M81, NL and MT are A-type viruses and AG876 and P3HR-1 (not shown but with gp340 sequence identical to AG876) are B-type. The prototype B95-8 sequence is shown in full as the top line of the comparison. In the other strains, invariant amino acids are indicated by a dot (.) and deleted residues appear as asterisks (*). The region spliced out of gp340 to form gp220 is between the square brackets [ ] above the B95-8 sequence.

lymphoma-induction model, which to some extent parallels post-transplant lymphoma in humans (see Section 4.8.4), a vaccine based on gp340/220 had the appropriate potential. The EBV gp340/220 coding sequences have been incorporated into several different live virus recombinant delivery systems with various degrees of subsequent characterization. The first approach utilized a vaccine strain of varicella zoster virus as a carrier. This virus has been extensively used in humans and has an acceptable safety record. However, although appropriate expression of gp340/220 has been obtained [58], the potential of this route has not been pursued.

The second system used adenoviruses which are currently finding an increasing role as vectors of foreign genes for gene therapy or as potential vaccines. Vaccination using a trivalent (serotypes 4, 7 and 21) adenovirus vaccine has been used extensively in the USA armed forces for the prevention of respiratory disease. The preparation appears to be effective and safe. A replication-defective adenovirus type 5 recombinant which expresses EBV gp340/220 has been constructed. This recombinant induces anti-MA antibodies following vaccination of rabbits and confers protection against EBV challenge in the cottontop tamarin model [59].

The recombinant adenovirus approach is attractive because of the feasibility of oral administration and the possibility of the development of oral, secretory antibodies due to the disposition of adenovirus to infect the tonsils and salivary glands. Production of such oral, secretory, neutralizing antibodies has often been considered to be potentially advantageous in combatting EBV whose primary route of transmission is oral. However, observations [60] suggest that EBV-specific secretory IgA may afford EBV with a means of infecting epithelial cells and, particularly if the antibodies do not neutralize virus, may enhance rather than inhibit virus infectivity; precisely opposite to the intended effect.

Third, incorporation of the gp340 gene into vaccinia virus recombinants resulted in the production of gp340 (vaccinia does not have an RNA splicing mechanism and therefore cannot produce gp220) which was highly glycosylated, could be detected on the cell surface of infected cells and had a molecular weight of about 340 kDa, all of which are properties of the authentic gp340 [61]. Sera from rabbits immunized with the recombinants neutralized EBV in a cord blood immortalization assay and, using a recombinant based on the virulent laboratory WR strain of vaccinia, protected cottontop tamarins in the challenge assay [62]. Interestingly, the protected animals did not possess any detectable serum antibodies against gp340, suggesting that the principal protective mechanism may be via cell-mediated rather than humoral responses.

More recently, Gu *et al.* [63] reported the construction of a similar recombinant virus using the Chinese vaccine strain of vaccinia, Tian Tan. The recombinant was shown to express a product which was recognized in tissue culture by sera from nasopharyngeal carcinoma (NPC) patients and when injected into rabbits raised antisera which reacted with the surface of B95-8 cells. The recombinant has subsequently been used in a small-scale trial in groups of adults and children. An appropriate anti-MA antibody response was generated in children who were serologically MA-negative prior to vaccination. Following this, a group of nine infants were vaccinated. Of these, three seroconverted via natural infection within 16 months, the other six remained EBV seronegative. Ten unvaccinated control infants all seroconverted within the same time period [64]. This small trial supports the concept that a vaccine based on gp340 alone will be protective in humans.

Recombinant vaccinia- or other poxviruses afford a simple and precedented (in the form of 'straight' vaccinia) means of mass vaccination. They are cheap to produce and therefore relatively affordable by developing countries with large target populations. In addition they have excellent potential as polyvalent vaccines due to their high capacity to accommodate additional DNA. An obvious example would be a joint EBV and HBV vaccine to tackle NPC and HCC, which between them account for about one-fifth to one-quarter of cancers in southern China (*Figure 7.1*). Unfortunately the advent of HIV infection in a significant proportion of the world population reduces the attractiveness of any live vaccine approach. For example, it is well-known that complications due to disseminated vaccinia occur at a much higher frequency in subjects who are in any way immunocompromized. For this reason a subunit vaccine may well be preferable.

### 7.5.4 A potential subunit vaccine

It is obvious that the yields of authentic gp340/220 that can be obtained from currently available EBV-carrying cell lines are woefully inadequate for any large-scale vaccine intervention initiative such as may be required in south-east Asia as a putative anti-NPC measure. In addition, even to achieve these levels, the potentially oncogenic phorbol ester 12-O-tetradecanoyl-phorbol-13-acetate (TPA) must be added to the cell cultures as an inducing agent, a compound which is unacceptable to the regulatory authorities. Omission of this inducer would reduce the already low levels by an order of magnitude. In order to overcome this problem, several laboratories have used a variety of genetic manipulation techniques in efforts to produce a biologically relevant, recombinant gp340/220 in viable amounts. Attempts using *Escherichia coli*, baculovirus or the yeasts *Saccharomyces cerevisiae* and *Pichia pastoris* were all, for a variety of reasons, unsuccessful in generating suitable products. Expression systems in cultured mammalian cells have greater potential to yield authentic products due to their capacity to perform appropriate post-translational modifications and several attempts at gp340/220 expression have been reported. Currently at least two mammalian cell lines are under serious study as potential sources of material on which to base a subunit vaccine. The first uses an expression plasmid driven by the SV40 early promoter and dehydrofolate reductase selection in a CHO cell line [65]. The second system drives gp340 /220 expression using the mouse metallothionine gene promoter carried in a vector in mouse C127 cells [66]. In both cases the levels of expression which are obtained are adequate for at least trial-size batches of material and may even be sufficient for full-scale production purposes.

Characterization of the product from the C127 system indicates that it appears to be of similar size (i.e. is probably similarly glycosylated) to the authentic proteins and raises virus-neutralizing antibodies in experimental animals. It is also recognized by human EBV-specific T cells (*Figure 7.8*) and is protective in the cottontop tamarin challenge system (*Figure 7.9*). Thus, the recombinant product appears to mirror the properties of the authentic antigen in many respects.

### 7.5.5 Other antigens

In many instances, cell-mediated immune responses are believed to be of crucial importance in vaccine effectiveness. The latent gene products EBNA2, EBNA3a, 3b, 3c and LMP have been shown to be targets for cytotoxic T cells

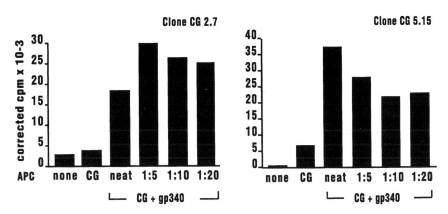

**Figure 7.8.** Proliferation of T-cell clones in response to purified gp340/220. Recognition of gp340/220 by clones CG2.7 and CG5.15 [67] is expressed as proliferation of each clone to different concentrations of gp340/220 in the presence of autologous LCL antigen presenting cells (APCs). Concentrations refer to the dilution of antigen present during the initial incubation with APCs (neat = 20 μg ml$^{-1}$). Reprinted from Vaccine volume 10, Madej *et al*, 1992, p.780, with permission from Elsevier Science.

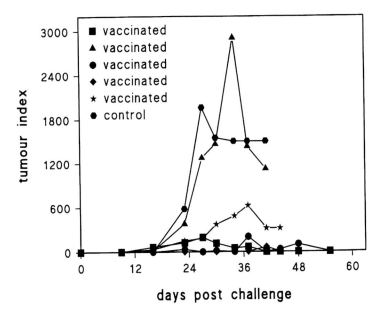

**Figure 7.9.** EBV challenge experiment in tamarins. Animals were vaccinated with recombinant gp340/220 in alhydrogel adjuvant (vaccinated) or with adjuvant alone (control). They were subsequently challenged with a tumorigenic dose of EBV. Tumour index is the sum of the volumes of palpable tumours in mm³.

involved in the virus–host balance and several CTL epitopes have been mapped precisely (see Section 4.6). Thus, some or all of these latent proteins could be considered as vaccine candidates which would generate specific CTLs against latently infected cells. Since several of these gene products are involved in EBV-mediated cellular immortalization (see Section 4.7) the use of the intact proteins as vaccine antigens would not be favoured. However, this problem can be overcome by using short peptides consisting of only the CTL epitope as immunogen. As mentioned in Section 7.4.4, immunization of mice with epitope peptides from HPV proteins has been shown to elicit an appropriate CTL response. Such a vaccine has the advantages of being completely synthetic and therefore free from the batch-to-batch biological variation which can occur with cell-derived products. A human trial is currently under way in Australia for the evaluation of the HLA B8 restricted epitope of EBNA 3a, FLRGRAYGL [68].

It is obvious from the discussion of EBV-specific CTL (Section 4.6) that many different peptides will be required in order to generate appropriate responses in the population as a whole, given the need to encompass the variety of susceptible targets dictated by HLA type, EBV type (A or B) and virus variation. Although the major CTL epitopes have been described (*Table 4.2*) the definition of the complete array of potential target epitopes requires more effort.

Delivery of the complete array of epitopes could be achieved simply by mixing peptides. However, it has been shown that a synthetic polyepitope delivered and expressed by recombinant vaccinia virus is effective in eliciting appropriate presentation of each individual epitope by its restricting allele [68].

### 7.5.6 Immediate prospects

The small trial using gp340-vaccinia is encouraging in so far as it suggests that a vaccine based on EBV MA may prevent primary infection. Attempts are currently being made to initiate human trials using a vaccine formulated using purified glycoprotein. It is likely that such trials will be carried out in a western population group of seronegatives and will assay for prevention of seroconversion and infectious mononucleosis (IM). Such a trial should produce meaningful results on a fairly short (3–5 year) timescale. The indications from both the vaccinia trial in China and the tamarin protection data imply that this type of vaccine should be effective at least in the prevention of IM since it ought to reduce the dose level of infecting virus. Whether such a vaccine will be effective in preventing EBV-associated cancer is debatable. It can be argued that in order to achieve such an end one must induce sterile immunity, that is the complete protection of infection and establishment of latency, and that this may not be attainable.

Trials using peptides to generate CTL responses have recently begun. This type of approach should be effective against both IM and immunoblastic lymphomas.

Assuming that the currently envisaged trials are successful, one can envisage moving on to further trials to assess the effect on EBV-associated cancer. Here the timescale is much longer. It will take at least 10 years to monitor an effect against Burkitt's lymphoma (peak incidence around 7 years of age) and at least 50 years for NPC. Nevertheless the potential benefits are enormous.

## 7.6 Human T-cell leukaemia virus type I vaccines

### 7.6.1 Introduction

Similar reservations to those raised against the feasibility of mass vaccination against HBV and EBV are frequently voiced in the context of human T-cell leukaemia virus type I (HTLV-I). Given the long latency between infection and the development of disease, particularly of adult T-cell leukaemia (ATL), a successful vaccination campaign might not be seen to reap benefit for a generation. It is difficult to predict whether vaccination of an already infected subject, perhaps better described as immunotherapy, would modify, abort or even precipitate disease, particularly if an apparently appropriate immune response is important in the pathogenesis of the inflammatory conditions. The majority of the target population live in the developing world, where other health concerns may have prior call on sparse resources.

Many of these concerns have their foundation in the harsh reality of commerce. Vaccines are produced by pharmaceutical companies who need to profit from their investment. If the return does not seem assured, the project does not proceed.

### 7.6.2 Target population

An estimated 15–20 million persons worldwide are infected with HTLV-I. Possible targets for vaccination would be the children of mothers known to have HTLV-I, particularly in situations where breast feeding rather than bottle feeding was desirable. In Japan, a project to identify and inform infected mothers of the risk of transmission of HTLV-I by breast feeding reduced the mother-to-child transmission rate from 25% to about 5% [69]. More recent data indicate that transmission due to breast feeding may not become significant unless breast feeding continues after 6 months of age [70]. Thus, there seems to be a 'window period' which is ideal either for active or passive immunization of the 'at risk' infant. However this type of health policy would require antenatal (or possibly even postnatal) testing. With the exception of Japan most communities which have the resources do not routinely screen for HTLV-I/II infection, indeed in Europe very little is known about the prevalence of HTLV-I/II among pregnant women [71]. Other groups who might be targeted are the partners of HTLV-I/II-infected subjects or high-risk groups such as intravenous drug users, commercial sex workers or those likely to require sequential polytransfusion. HTLV-I/II infection, along with other parenteral infections, for example HIV, HBV or HCV could, however, be prevented in some of these groups by more generalized measures: education; needle-exchange programmes; safer-sex practices; condom use; screening of donated blood.

### 7.6.3 Envelope glycoproteins

The envelope glycoproteins of retroviruses interact with cell surface receptors during infection of target cells and play a major role in eliciting host antiviral immunity [72]. The Env proteins of animal retroviruses will induce humoral immunity which protects the host against viral infection [73,74]. *In vitro* experiments have indicated that anti-HTLV-I Env glycoprotein, gp46, should be similarly protective [75] and could form the basis of an effective vaccine. This rationale is similar to that applied to HBV (see Section 7.2.1) and EBV (see Section 7.5.2).

That antibodies can protect against mucosal exposure to HTLV-I is indicated by the lack of transmission of HTLV-I to the breast fed offspring of infected mothers during the first 6 months of breast feeding compared with the linear rise in infection rates thereafter [76] which coincides with declining maternal antibody. This has been confirmed in the rabbit model where immunization with immunoglobulin has been shown to protect against both blood transfusion [77] and milk-borne [78] transmission of HTLV-I.

Given the lack of intra-isolate diversity [79] (see Section 6.3.2 and *Figure 6.4*) a vaccine, based on the *env* gene product, to prevent infection appears more easily attainable for HTLV-I and HTLV-II than for the more pressing HIV.

### 7.6.4 Experimental vaccines

Studies of active vaccination against HTLV-I and HTLV-II have been conducted in a number of animal models with a variety of vaccines, many of which are live recombinant virus-based. A number of inbred species of rat (Fischer F344, Lewis and Brown Norway) can be infected with HTLV-I to a low level. The induction of Env antibodies and partial protection against HTLV-I infection was induced by *env*–vaccinia and *env*–adenovirus recombinant vaccines [80].

Rabbits were protected against HTLV-I by an *env*–vaccinia recombinant vaccine [81] when challenged with MT-2 cells, a transformed human cell line. Similarly an *env*–avipox virus recombinant was able to protect rabbits challenged with HTLV-I-infected human cells, but did not protect against HTLV-I-infected rabbit cells [82] suggesting that anti-HLA antibodies or cellular immunity might enhance the protective effect. This would appear to be analogous to the situation seen in HIV [83]. Rabbits can also be protected against HTLV-II using recombinant precursor protein gp63, with production of both of the *env* products gp46 (which induces neutralizing antibodies) and gp21 (important in cell fusion and thus in cell-to-cell transmission) – ligated into a baculovirus and propagated in insect cells. The protected rabbits were challenged 4 weeks after the third vaccination with an intravenous inoculation of a human HTLV-II cell line [84].

Protein subunit vaccines have been tested in two species of macaque, the pigtailed (*Macaca nemestrina*) and cynomolgus (*Macaca fascicularis*). Pigtailed macaques were protected from challenge with STLV-I by soluble HTLV-I proteins [85], whilst the cynomolgus monkeys were protected from HTLV-I by inoculation with recombinant Env proteins expressed in *E. coli* [86].

### 7.6.5 Potential trials

It has been pointed out that because the target populations are located primarily in developing countries, the vaccine needs to be cheap and should preferably be suitable for oral administration. On this basis it was suggested that the live recombinant defective adenovirus approach would be appropriate [87]. A suitable target population for initial trials could be children of HTLV-I-positive mothers. Epidemiological studies have been initiated in order to identify a suitable trial population [87].

## 7.7 Viral therapy of human cancer

### 7.7.1 Introduction

Alongside efforts to develop preventive anticancer vaccines (prophylaxis), there are a range of approaches to virus-based methods under investigation for the treatment of cancers (therapy) (*Table 7.1*). Some of these are directed towards virally-induced cancers and are closely related to the vaccines under development. These may even use the same vaccine-based approach. A good example of this is studies of the therapeutic use of a candidate papillomavirus vaccine based on a recombinant vaccinia virus (see Section 7.4.6). In this

**Table 7.1.** Virus-mediated anticancer therapies

| Strategy | Example |
|---|---|
| Vaccine-based immunotherapy[a] | Recombinant vaccinia virus expressing papillomavirus antigens |
| Heterologous virus immunostimulation[a] | Treatment with cancer cells infected with avian paramyxovirus (NDV) |
| Direct cell killing[b] | Mutated adenovirus lacking E1B p53 inhibitor (only able to grow in those cells, usually tumour cells, lacking this function) |
| Genetically enhanced immune mediated cell killing[b] | Recombinant vaccinia virus expressing B7 co-stimulatory protein |
| Virus-directed enzyme/ prodrug therapy (VDEPT)[b] | Recombinant adenovirus expressing herpes simplex virus thymidine kinase (HSVtk) gene, combined with systemic treatment with ganciclovir (prodrug requiring activation by HSVtk) |
| Expression of cytokine gene[b] | Recombinant adenovirus expressing interferon gene |
| Antisense inhibition of protein sustaining malignant tumour cell phenotype[b] | Recombinant adenovirus expressing antisense insulin-like growth factor I receptor |
| Protection of vulnerable cells from effects of anticancer drugs[c] | Expression of O-6-methylguanine-DNA methyltransferase gene in haematopoietic stem cells (protects against alkylating agents) |

[a] Systemic administration.
[b] Direct administration to tumour (improved targeting systems may allow systemic administration).
[c] Direct administration to target (non-tumour) cells which are to be protected (improved targeting systems may allow systemic administration).
NDV, Newcastle disease virus.

study, the vaccine virus was administered to patients with late stage cervical cancer, and promising immune responses were observed in some cases [50].

### 7.7.2 Viruses as delivery vehicles

A common approach is the use of recombinant viruses as vectors to deliver genes with anticancer properties into the target cells. This is actually a specialized form of gene therapy. A widely used method is the introduction of a herpesvirus thymidine kinase gene, under the control of an appropriate promoter [88], which may be optimized for expression in tumour cells [89]. The gene product is in itself harmless, but renders the cell vulnerable to treatment with anti-herpesvirus nucleoside analogue drugs such as acyclovir [9-(2-hydroxyethoxymethyl) guanine] or ganciclovir [9-(1,3-dihydroxy-2-propoxymethyl) guanine]. These drugs, which are widely used to treat herpesvirus infections, are not toxic to normal cells since they are precursors of the active form of the drug (prodrugs), and require activation by the viral thymidine kinase gene. However, if this gene is expressed in cells, either due to virus infection or as part of anti-cancer therapy, the nucleoside analogue is activated by phosphorylation, allowing it to disrupt DNA synthesis and prevent replication of the cell [90,91]. This is referred to as VDEPT (virus-directed enzyme/prodrug therapy) and is a variation of the related ADEPT strategy where antibody attached to an enzyme is used to direct it to a tumour where it can convert the prodrug to an active form.

Most work with VDEPT has used recombinant adenoviruses to carry the thymidine kinase gene from herpes simplex virus, combined with administration of ganciclovir. While most work has to date used model systems, promising results have been obtained [92], and a clinical study has been described [93]. One interesting effect that may increase the effectiveness of VDEPT is that surrounding 'bystander' cells which do not express the thymidine kinase gene may also be killed following drug treatment, apparently by the induction of apoptosis [94]. This has the potential to increase the localized cytocidal effect of the treatment, enhancing its tumour-killing effect.

Alternatively, viral vectors may be used to introduce genes which exert a direct antiviral or immunostimulatory effect, such as those for interferon [95] or interleukins [96,97]. Virus-mediated expression of immune co-stimulators such as the B7 molecule [98] may enhance activation of T cells and thus potentiate the immune response, in contrast to the direct cytocidal effects of VDEPT. Viral vectors have also been used to introduce antisense molecules inhibiting viral transforming genes [99], cellular genes associated with maintaining the cell in a malignant state [100,101], or other repressors of such genes [102]. The use of genes to stimulate apoptosis in tumour cells has also been suggested [103]. In some systems, virus-derived plasmids may be used to deliver genes to tumour cells by using systems other than whole virus, such as fusogenic liposomes [104].

An alternative approach uses viral vectors to increase drug resistance in normal cells which are vulnerable to the chemotherapeutic drugs used to treat cancers [105]. In studies with haematopoietic stem cells [106], the viral vector carries a gene which makes the cells resistant to the toxic effects of alkylating agents, allowing the use of higher levels of these drugs against the cancer.

### 7.7.3 Targeting

The principal aim of cancer therapy is to annihilate the tumour cells whilst maintaining the surrounding cells normal and unharmed. Therefore much effort is being expended in devising strategies of viral delivery which fulfil this objective. One interesting development relies on removing a viral gene, rather than adding an extra gene as in the approaches described above. In this system, a modified adenovirus is used which is cytopathic only for tumour cells [107]. This virus lacks the viral E1B gene, which is required for adenovirus replication in normal cells. The function of the E1B protein is to inactivate the cellular p53 protein, an important tumour suppressor protein concerned with controlling apoptosis. The function of p53 is commonly inhibited in cancer cells (see Sections 1.6, 2.7.2, 3.5.2 and 6.5.9), and it is only in cells where it is inactivated that the mutated virus can replicate and kill the cell. Thus, the mutated virus preferentially kills cancer cells.

Other studies are based on the natural tropism of a particular virus. Some efforts used avirulent strains of an avian Paramyxovirus, Newcastle disease virus (fowl pest, NDV) which was able to infect and kill human cancer cells but appeared less able to infect normal human cells (although NDV conjunctivitis is known in laboratory workers). NDV was also used to recruit immunological mechanisms to target the malignant cells [108–112]. These investigations involved both animal studies and clinical trials, and promising results were obtained. Earlier work used the related mumps Paramyxovirus to enhance the immune response [113,114], but there are problems with any approach using a live human pathogen in immunosuppressed patients (see Section 7.5.3).

In the studies outlined above, a wide range of viral vectors has been evaluated (*Table 7.2*), including adenoviruses, herpesviruses, papovaviruses (papillomavirus), parvoviruses (adeno-associated virus), poxviruses (vaccinia), and retroviruses. In most cases, virus is administered by direct injection into the tumour body. While this may prove effective in model systems, in clinical applications this is likely to be more difficult since the tumour may be inaccessible. In addition, such methods will not treat metastasized (secondary) tumours. Ideally, systemic administration would be used, allowing migration of the virus around the body. This would permit infection of tumour cells in multiple locations. However, this is likely to require highly specific viruses which infect only the target (tumour) cells, since many different cell types would be exposed to the virus. Some animal retroviruses can show high tissue specificity, for example murine mammary tumour virus in a breast cancer model ([100] and systemic administration has

**Table 7.2.** Viral vector systems used for anticancer therapies

| Virus | Advantages | Disadvantages |
|-------|------------|---------------|
| Adenoviruses (*Adenoviridae*) | Large genome (30–38 kb) allows large inserts (7 kb possible); can be administered via respiratory route (if targeting systems developed) | Could be spread by aerosol; viral DNA does not integrate efficiently; may be oncogenic |
| Herpes simplex virus (*Herpesviridae*) | Very large genome (152 kb) allows large inserts (10 kb possible, even larger in some systems); viral DNA can be maintained as stable extrachromosomal element (episome); virus can mediate entry into central nervous system | Most genes may be inactive in episomal state; may be pathogenic or oncogenic |
| Papillomavirus (*Papovaviridae*) | Persistent (episomal) infection may be established; virus can target neuronal cells | Small genome (7.5 kb total) restricts insert size; may be oncogenic |
| Adeno-associated virus (*Parvoviridae*) | Efficient integration at specific site; non-pathogenic | Very small genome (5 kb total) severely restricts insert size |
| Vaccinia virus (*Poxviridae*) | Very large genome (192 kb) allows very large inserts (25 kb possible) | No persistent state, viral genome does not integrate; may be pathogenic |
| Retroviruses (*Retroviridae*) | High efficiency integration (at variable sites); very specific cell types infected by individual viruses | Small genome (7–10kb total) restricts insert size; high mutation rate; may be oncogenic |

been used in clinical studies with NDV, see above). However, it is probable that in future studies the specificity of recombinant viruses will be increased by inserting specific receptor molecules into the viral surface. This approach is similar to that used in ADEPT, where antibody–drug conjugates are constructed that will bind preferentially to tumour cells, using antibodies to unusual surface molecules expressed on the tumour cells. Indeed, the construction of antibody–virus hybrids ('immunoviruses') has been suggested as a way to achieve the necessary specificity [115].

## 7.7.4 Outlook

It is important to note that, despite all of the work described above, viral therapy for cancer is at best in early trials, and it is unlikely that such approaches will be in widespread use for many years. In particular, targeting the virus to the tumour and ensuring that the virus is not pathogenic even in profoundly immunosuppressed individuals will be very important. However, promising approaches have been identified and are under active investigation.

## References

1. **Muir, C., Waterhouse, J. Mack, T., Powell, J. and Whelan, S.** (eds). (1987) *Cancer Incidence in Five Continents.* Vol. V. IARC Scientific Publication 88. International Agency for Research on Cancer, Lyon.
2. **McAuliffe, V.J., Purcell, R.H. and Gerin, J.L.** (1980) *Rev. Infect. Dis.* **2:** 470–492..
3. **Hilleman, M.R.** (1993) in *Hepatitis B Vaccines in Clinical Practice.* (ed. R.W. Ellis). Marcel Dekker Inc., New York, pp.17–39.
4. **Poovorawan, Y., Sanpavat, S., Pongpunlert, W., Chumdermpadetsuk, S., Sentrakul, P., Chitinand, S., Sakulramrung, R. and Tannirundorn, Y.** (1990) *Vaccine* **8:** S56–S59.
5. **Andre, F.E. and Zuckerman, A.J.** (1994) *J. Med. Virol.* **44:** 144–151.
6. **Stirk, H.J., Thornton, J.M. and Howard, C.R.** (1992) *Intervirology* **33:** 148–158.
7. **Coberly, J.S., Townsend, T., Repke, J., Fields, H., Margolis, H. and Halsey, N.A.** (1994) *Vaccine* **12:** 984–987.
8. **Milich, D.R.** (1988) *Immunol. Today* **9:** 380–386.
9. **Carman, W.F., Zanetti, A.R., Karayiannis, P., Waters, J., Manzillo, G., Tanzi, E., Zuckerman, A.J. and Thomas, H.C.** (1990) *Lancet,* **336:** 325–329.
10. **Harrison, T.J., Hopes, E.A., Oon, C.J, Zanetti, A.R. and Zuckerman, A.J.** (1991) *J. Hepatol.,* **13:** S105–S107.
11. **Fujii, H., Moriyama, K., Sakamoto, N., Kondo, T., Yasuda, K., Hiraizumi, Y., Yamazaki, M., Sakaki, Y., Okochi, K. and Nakajima, E.** (1992) *Biochem. Biophys. Res. Comm.* **184:** 1152–1157.
12. **Yamamoto, K., Horikita, M., Tsuda, F., Itoh, K., Akahane, Y., Yotsumoto, S., Okamoto, H., Miyakawa, Y. and Mayumi, M.** (1994) *J. Virol.* **68:** 2671–2676.
13. **Oon, C.-J., Lim, G.-K., Ye, Z., Goh, K.-T., Tan, K.-L., Yo, S.-L., Hopes, E., Harrison, T.J. and Zuckerman A.J.** (1995) *Vaccine* **13:** 699–702.
14. **Karthigesu, V.D., Allison, L.M.C., Fortuin, M., Mendy, M., Whittle, H.C. and Howard, C.R.** (1994) *J. Gen. Virol.* **75:** 443–448.
15. **Harrison, T.J., Oon, C.J. and Zuckerman, A.J.** (1994) in *Viral Hepatitis and Liver Disease.* (eds K. Nishioka, H. Suzuki, S. Mishiro and T. Oda). Springer-Verlag, Tokyo, pp.248–251.
16. **McMahon, G., Ehrlich, P.H., Moustafa, Z.A., McCarthy, L.A., Dottavio, D., Tolpin, M.D., Nadler, P.I. and Ostberg, L.** (1992) *Hepatology* **15:** 757–766.
17. **Waters, J.A., Kennedy, M., Voet, P., Hauser, P., Petre, J., Carman, W. and Thomas, H.C.** (1992) *J. Clin. Invest.* **90:** 2543.
18. **Wong, V.C., Ip, H.M., Reesink, H.W., Lelie, P.N., Reerink-Brongers, E.E. and Yeung, C.Y.** (1984) *Lancet* i: 921–926.
19. **Del Canho, R., Grosheide, P.M., Schalm, S.W., de Vries, R.R. and Heijtink, R.A.** (1994) *J. Hepatol.* **20:** 483–486.
20. **Neurath, A.R., Kent, S.B. and Strick N.** (1986) *J. Gen. Virol.* **67:** 453–461.
21. **Tron, F., Degos, F., Brechot, C. et al.** (1989) *J. Infect. Dis.* **160:** 199–204.

22. **Shouval, D., Ilan, Y., Hourvitz, A.** *et al.* (1994) in *Viral Hepatitis and Liver Disease.* (eds K. Nishioka, H. Suzuki, S. Mishiro, T. Oda). Springer-Verlag, Tokyo, pp. 543–546.
23. **Zuckerman, J.N., Sabin, C., Craig, F.M., Williams, A. and Zuckerman, A.J.** (1997) *Br. Med. J.* **314:** 329–333.
24. **Alter M.J., Shapiro, C.N., Coleman, P.J. and Margolis, H.S.** (1994) in *Viral Hepatitis and Liver Disease.* (eds K. Nishioka, H. Suzuki, S. Mishiro, T. Oda). Springer-Verlag, Tokyo, pp.439–443.
25. **Chang, M.H., Chen, C.J., Lai, M.S., Hsu, H.M., Wu, T.C., Kong, M.S., Liang, D.C., Shau, W.Y. and Chen, D.S.** (1997) *New Engl. J. Med.* **336:** 1855–1959.
26. **Choo Q.L., Kuo, G., Weiner, A.J., Overby, L.R., Bradley, D.W. and Houghton, M.** (1989) *Science* **244:** 359–362.
27. **Kuo, G, Choo, Q.L., Alter, H.J.** *et al.* (1989). *Science* **244:** 362–364.
28. **Lesniewski, R.R., Boardway, K.M., Casey, J.M., Desai, S.M., Devare, S.G., Leung, T.K. and Mushahwar, I.K.** (1993) *J. Med. Virol* **40:** 150–156.
29. **Farci, P., Alter, H.J., Govindarajan, S., Wong, D.C., Engle, R., Lesniewski, R.R., Mushahwar, I.K., Desai, S.M., Miller, R.H., Ogata, N. and Purcell, R.H.** (1992) *Science* **258:** 135–140.
30. **Weiner, A.J., Geysen, H.M., Christopherson, C.** *et al.* (1992) *Proc. Natl Acad. Sci. USA* **89:** 3468–3472.
31. **Choo, Q.L., Kuo, G., Ralston, R.** *et al.* (1994) *Proc. Natl Acad. Sci. USA* **91:** 1294–1298.
32. **Murray, K., Bruce, S.A., Hinnen, A., Wingfield, P., van Erd, P.M. and de Reus, A.** (1984) *EMBO J.* **3:** 645–650.
33. **Murray, K., Bruce, S.A., Wingfield, P., van Erd, P.M., de Reus, A. and Schellekens, H.** (1987) *J. Med. Virol.* **23:** 101–107.
34. **Seeff, L.B., Alter, H.J.** (1994) *Ann. Intern. Med.* **120:** 807–809.
35. **Zuckerman, J., Clewley, G., Griffiths, P. and Cockroft, A.** (1994) *Lancet* **343:** 1618–1620.
36. **McMichael, A.J. and Bodmer, W.F.** (eds) (1992). *A New Look at Tumour Immunology. Cancer Surveys* 13. Cold Spring Harbor Laboratory Press, New York.
37. **Bodmer, W.F. and Owen, M.J.** (eds) (1995). *Molecular Mechanisms of the Immune Response. Cancer Surveys* **22:** Cold Spring Harbor Laboratory Press, New York.
38. **Kast, W.M., Roux, L., Curren, J, Blom, H.J.J., Voordouw, A.C., Meloen, R.H., Kolakofsky, D. and Melief, C.J.M.** (1991). *Proc. Natl Acad. Sci. USA,* **88:** 2283–2287.
39. **Kast, W.M., Brandt, R.M.P., Drijfhout, J.W. and Melief, C.J.M.** (1993) *J. Immunother.* **14:** 115–120.
40. **Bartholomew, J.S., Stacey, S.N., Coles, B., Burt, D.J., Arrand, J.R. and Stern, P.L.** (1994) *Eur. J. Immunol.* **24:** 3175–3179.
41. **Campo, M.S.** (1994). in *Human Papillomaviruses and Cervical Cancer: Biology and Immunology.* (eds. P.L. Stern and M.A. Stanley). *Oxford University Press,* Oxford, pp. 177–191.
42. **Feltkamp, M.C.W., Smits, H.L., Vierboom, M.P.M., Minnaar, R.P., DeJongh, B.M., Drijfhout, J.W., TerSchegget, J., Melief, C.J.M. and Kast, W.M.** (1993) *Eur. J. Immunol.* **23:** 2241–2249.
43. **Chen, L., Thomas, E.K., Hu, S.L., Hellstrom, I. and Hellstrom, K.E.** (1991) *Proc. Natl Acad.Sci. USA* **88:** 110–114.

44. **Beverley, P.C.L., Sadovnikova, E., Zhu, X., Hickling, J., Gao, L., Chain, B., Collins, S., Crawford, L., Vousden, K. and Stauss, H.J.** (1994) in *Vaccines Against Virally Induced Cancers.* Ciba Foundation Symposium 187. John Wiley & Sons, Chichester, pp. 78–86.

45. **Christensen, N.D., Kirnbauer, R., Schiller, J.T., Ghim, S.-J., Schlegel, R., Jenson, A.B. and Kreider, J.W.** (1994) *Virology* **205:** 329–335.

46. **Rose, R.C., Reichman, R.C. and Bonnez, W.** (1994) *J. Gen. Virol.* **75:** 2075–2079.

47. **Rose, R.C., Bonnez, W., Da Rin, C., McCance, D.J. and Reichman, R.C.** (1994) *J. Gen. Virol.* **75:** 2445–2449.

48. **Christensen, N.D., Reed, C.A., Cladel, N.M., Han, R. and Kreider, J.W.** (1996) *J. Virol.* **70:** 960–965.

49. **Suzich, J.A., Ghim, S.J., Palmer-Hill, F.J., White, W.I., Tamura, J.K., Bell, J. A., Newsome, J.A., Jenson, A.B. and Schlegel, R.** (1995) *Proc. Natl Acad. Sci. USA* **92:** 11553–11557.

50. **Borysiewicz, L.K., Fiander, A., Nimako, M. et al.** (1996). *Lancet* **347:** 1523–1527.

51. **Schiller, J. T. and Okun, M.** (1996) *Adv. Dermatol.* **11:** 355–380.

52. **Stern, P.L. and Duggan-Keen, M.F.** (1994). in *Human Papillomaviruses and Cervical Cancer: Biology and Immunology.* (eds. P.L. Stern and M.A. Stanley). Oxford University Press, Oxford, pp. 162–176

53. **Ellis, J.R.M., Keating, P.J., Baird, J. et al.** (1995). *Nature Med.* **1:** 464–470.

54. **Epstein, M.A.** (1976). *J. Natl Cancer. Inst.* **56:** 697–700.

55. **Arrand, J.R.** (1992). The Cancer Journal **5:** 188–193. Updated version on the Internet at http://www.infobiogen.fr/agora/journals/cancer/articles/5-4/arra.htm

56. **Lees, J.F., Arrand, J.E., Pepper, S. deV., Stewart, J.P., Mackett, M. and Arrand, J.R.** (1993). *Virology* **195:** 578–586.

57. **Epstein, M.A. and Achong, B.G.** (eds), (1986). *The Epstein Barr Virus: Recent Advances.* William Heineman Books, London.

58. **Lowe, R.S., Keller, P.M., Keech, B.J., Davison, A.J., Whang, Y., Morgan, A.J., Kieff, E. and Ellis R.W.** (1987) *Proc. Natl Acad. Sci. USA* **84:** 3893–3900.

59. **Ragot, T., Finerty, S., Watkins, P.E., Perricaudet, M. and Morgan, A.J.** (1993) *J. Gen .Virol.* **74:** 501–507.

60. **Sixbey, J.W. and Yao, Q.-Y.** (1992) *Science* **255:** 1578–1580.

61. **Mackett, M. and Arrand, J.R.** (1985). *EMBO J.* **4:** 3229–3234.

62. **Morgan, A.J., Mackett, M., Finerty, S., Arrand, J.R. and Epstein, M.A.** (1988) *J. Med. Virol.* **25:** 189–196.

63. **Gu, S., Huang, T., Miao, Y., Ruan, L., Zhao, Y., Han, C., Xiao, Y., Zhu, J. and Wolf, H.** (1991) *Chinese Med. Sci. J.* **6:** 241–243.

64. **Gu, S.Y., Huang, T.M., Ruan, L., Miao, Y.H., Lu, H., Chu, C.M., Motz, M. and Wolf, H.** (1993) in *The Epstein-Barr Virus and Associated Diseases.* (eds T. Tursz, J.S. Pagano, D.V. Ablashi, G. de Thé, G. Lenoir and G. Pearson). John Libbey Eurotext, Paris, pp. 579–584.

65. **Motz, M., Deby, G., and Wolf, H.** (1987). *Gene* **58:**149–154.

66. **Madej, M., Conway, M.J., Morgan, A.J., Sweet, J., Wallace L., Qualtiere, L.F., Arrand, J.R. and Mackett M.** (1992) *Vaccine* **10:** 777–782.

67. **Wallace, L.E., Wright, J., Uleato, D.O., Morgan, A.J. and Rickinson, A.B.** (1991) *J. Virol.* **65:** 3821–3828.

68. **Moss, D.J., Burrows, S.R., Suhrbier, A. and Khanna, R.** (1994). in *Vaccines Against Virally Induced Cancers.* Ciba Foundation Symposium 187. John Wiley & Sons, Chichester, pp. 4–13.

69. Hino, S., Sugiyama, H., Doi, H., Ishimaru T., Yamabe T., Tsuji Y. and Miyamoto, T. (1987) *Lancet* ii: 158–159.
70. Takezaki T., Tajima K., Ito, M., Ito, S.-I., Kinoshita, K.-I., Tachibana, K. and Matsushita, Y. (1997). *Leukaemia* 11: (Ssuppl.3) 60–62.
71. The HTLV European Research Network (1996). *Acquir. Immune Defic. Syndr. Hum. Retrovirol.* 13: 68–77.
72. Dickson, C., Eisenman, R., Fan, F., Hunter, E. and Teich, N. (1982) *in RNA Tumour Viruses.* (eds R.A. Weiss, N. Teich, H. Varmus and J. Coffin). Cold Spring Harbor Laboratory, New York, pp. 513–616.
73. Kleiser, C., Schneider, J., Bayer, H. and Hunsmann, G. (1986). *J. Gen. Virol.* 67: 1901–1907.
74. Onuma, M., Watarai, S., Mikami, T. and Izawa, H. (1984) *Am. J. Vet. Res.* 45: 1212–1215.
75. Hoshino, H., Clapham, P.R., Weiss, R.A., Miyoshi, I., Yoshida, M. and Miwa, M. (1985) *Int. J. Cancer* 36: 671–675.
76. Takahashi, K., Takezaki, T., Oki, T. *et al.* (1991). *Int J. Cancer* 49: 673–677.
77. Kataoka, R., Takehara, N., Iwahara, Y., Sawada, T., Ohtsuki, Y., Dawei, Y., Hoshino, H. and Miyoshi, I. (1990) *Blood* 76: 1657–1661.
78. Sawada, T., Iwahara, Y., Ishii, K., Taguchi, H., Hoshino, H. and Miyoshi, I. (1991) *J. Infect. Dis.* 164: 1193–1196.
79. Liu, H.-F., Goubau, P., Van Brussel, M., Van Laethem, K., Chen, Y.-C., Desmyter, J. and Vandamme, A.-M. (1996). *J. Gen. Virol.* 77: 359–368.
80. Bomford, R., Kazanji, M. and de Thé G. (1996) *AIDS Res. Hum. Retroviruses* 12: 403–405.
81. Shida, M., Tachikura, T., Sato, T. *et al.* (1987). *EMBO J.* 6: 3379–3384.
82. Franchini, G., Tartaglia, J., Markham, P., Benson, J., Fullen, J., Wills, M., Arp, J., Dekaban, G., Paoletti, E. and Gallo, R.C. (1995) *AIDS Res. Hum. Retroviruses* 11: 30–313.
83. Stott, E.J. (1991) *Nature* 353: 393.
84. Hall, W.W. (1997) Presented at VIIIth International Conference on Human Retrovirology: HTLV, Rio de Janeiro, June 9–13.
85. Dezzuti, C.S., Frazier, F.E., Huff, L.Y., Stromberg, P.C. and Olsen, R.G. (1990) *Cancer Res.* 50: s5687–s5691.
86. Nakamura, H., Hayami, M., Ohta, Y., Ishikawa, K.-I., Tsujimoto, H., Kiyokawa, T., Yoshida, M., Sasagawa, A. and Honjo, S. (1987) *Int. J. Cancer* 40: 403–407.
87. de Thé, G., Bomford, R., Kazanji, M. and Ibrahim. F. (1994) in *Vaccines Against Virally Induced Cancers.* Ciba Foundation Symposium 187. John Wiley & Sons, Chichester, pp. 47–55.
88. Freeman, S.M. Whartenby, K.A., Freeman, J.L., Abboud, C.N. and Marrogi, A.J. (1996) *Sem. Oncol.* 23: 31–45.
89. Kumagai, T., Tanio, Y., Osaki, T., Hosoe, S., Tachibana, I., Ueno, K., Kijima, T., Horai, T. and Kishimoto, T. (1996) *Cancer Res.* 56: 354–358.
90. Black, M.E., Newcomb, T.G., Wilson, H.M. and Loeb, L.A. (1996). *Proc. Nat Acad. Sci.* USA 93: 3525–3529.
91. Hasegawa, Y., Emi, N. and Shimokata, K. (1995) *J. Mol. Med.* 73: 107–112.
92. Connors, T.A. and Knox, R.J. (1995). *Stem Cells* 13: 501–511.
93. Oldfield, E.H., Ram, Z., Culver, K.W., Blaese, R.M., DeVroom, H.L. and Anderson, W.F. (1993). *Hum. Gene Ther.* 4: 39–69.
94. Hamel, W., Magnelli, L., Chiarugi, V.P. and Israel, M.A. (1996). *Cancer Res.* 56: 2697–2702.

95.  Zhang, J.F., Hu, C., Geng, Y, Selm, J., Klein, S.B., Orazi, A. and Taylor, M,W. (1996) *Proc. Natl Acad. Sci. USA* **93**: 4513–4518.
96.  Whitman, E.D., Tsung, K., Paxson, J. and Norton, J.A. (1994). *Surgery* **116**: 183–188.
97.  Zitvogel, L., Tahara, H., Cai, Q., Storkus, W.J., Muller, G., Wolf, S.F., Gately, M., Robbins, P.D. and Lotze, M.T. (1994) *Hum. Gene Ther.* **5**: 1493–1506.
98.  Hodge, J.W., Abrams, S., Schlom, J. and Kantor, J.A. (1994) *Cancer Res.* **54**: 5552–5555.
99.  Hamada, K., Sakaue, M., Alemany, R., Zhang, W.W., Horio, Y., Roth, J.A. and Mitchell, M.F. (1996) *Gynecol. Oncol.* **63**: 219–227.
100.  Arteaga, C.L. and Holt, J.T. (1996) *Cancer Res.* **56**: 1098–1103.
101.  Lee, C.T., Wu, S., Gabrilovich, D., Chen, H., Nadaf-Rahrov, S., Cierni, I.F. and Carbone, D.P. (1996) *Cancer Res.* **56**: 3038–3041.
102.  Zhang, Y., Yu, D., Xia, W., Hung, M.C. (1995) *Oncogene* **10**: 1947–1954.
103.  Sinkovics, J.G. and Horvath, J. (1995) *Medical Hypotheses* **44**: 359–368 **45**: 316.
104.  Vieweg, J., Boczkowski, D., Roberson K.M., Edwards, D.W., Philip, M., Philip, R., Rudoll, T., Smith, C., Robertson, C. and Gilboa, E. (1995) *Cancer Res.* **55**: 2366–2372.
105.  Kelley, S.L., Basu, A., Teicher, B.A., Hacker, M.P., Hamer, D.H. and Lazo, J.S. (1988) *Science* **241**: 1813–1815.
106.  Wang, G., Weiss, C., Sheng, P. and Bresnick, E. (1996) *Biochem. Pharmacol.* **51**:1221–1228
107.  Bischoff, J.R., Kirn, D.H., Williams, A. *et al.* (1996) *Science* **274**: 373–376.
108.  Csatary, L.K., Eckhardt, S., Bukosza, I., Czegledi, F., Fenyvesi, C., Gergely, P., Bodey, B. and Csatary, C.M. (1993) *Cancer Detect. Prev.* **17 6**:19–627.
109.  Lehner, B., Schlag, P., Liebrich, W. and Schirrmacher, V. (1990) *Cancer Immunol. Immunother.* **32**: 173–178.
110.  Liebrich, W., Schlag, P., Manasterski, M., Lehner, B., Stohr, M., Moller, P. and Schirrmacher, V. (1991) *Eur. J. Cancer* **27**: 703–710.
111.  Lorence, R.M., Reichard, K.W., Katubig, B.B., Reyes, H.M., Phuangsab, A., Mitchell, B.R., Cascino, C.J., Walter, R.J. and Peeples, M.E. (1994) *J. Natl Cancer Ins.* **86**: 1228–1233.
112.  Schlag, P., Manasterski, M., Gerneth, T., Hohenberger, P., Dueck, M., Herfarth, C., Liebrich, W. and Schirrmacher, V. (1992) *Cancer Immunol. Immunother.* **35**: 325–330.
113.  Sato, M., Urade, M., Sakuda, M., Shirasuna, K., Yoshida, H., Maeda N., Yanagawa, T., Morimoto, M., Yura, Y., Miyazaki, T., Okuno, Y. and Takahashi, M. (1979) *Int. J. Oral Surg.* **8**: 205–211.
114.  Shimizu, Y., Hasumi, K., Okudaira, Y., Yamanishi, K. and Takahashi, M. (1988) *Cancer Detect. Prev.* **12**: 487–495
115.  Wawrzynczak, E.J. (1995) *Antibody Therapy*. Bios Scientific Publishers, Oxford.

## Further reading

Ellis, R.W. (1993) *Hepatitis B vaccines in Clinical Practice*. Marcel Dekker Inc., New York.

# Index